CANADIAN HOSPITALS, 1920 TO 1970

G. HARVEY AGNEW, MD, LLD, FACP, FACHA

Canadian Hospitals, 1920 to 1970
A Dramatic Half Century

UNIVERSITY OF TORONTO PRESS

©University of Toronto Press 1974
Toronto and Buffalo
Printed in Canada

ISBN 0-8020-1994-3
LC 73-78942

Contents

Foreword

For some years a group of friends had been pressing Harvey Agnew to write a book on the history of modern hospital development in Canada. However, pressure of work and other demands on his time prevented him from accepting the challenge until 1970 after he had officially retired.

He undertook this enormous task, like all others he tackled, with thoroughness and vigor. Every chapter was planned in detail long before the writing started. For this we are most fortunate indeed, because after his death it was possible for others to complete the work by following the original outline.

In this eagerly awaited book will be found the lessons learned over fifty years so that present and following generations of hospital people will not need to relearn them over and over again.

Only Harvey Agnew could have written this book. His extensive knowledge and penetrating insight allowed him, all through the years, to evaluate new methods, new developments, new concepts and to appreciate their long-range effect on hospital organization, administration and planning and the ultimate benefit to better patient care.

During this, the most important phase of hospital development in Canada, he witnessed and participated in the transformation of the hospital from a measure of last resort to the hub for the delivery of health care; he displays the whole panorama before us.

The importance of hospital associations in the development of hospitals was realized very early by Dr Agnew. In 1928 he left a promising career in medicine and teaching to take charge of the newly formed Department of Hospital Service of the Canadian Medical Association.

His long service with the Canadian Hospital Council, later the Canadian Hospital Association, put him in a vantage position to follow and influence the hospital scene in Canada. He has used the knowledge so gained to bring to us the intimate details of the evolution and progress of hospitals in this country.

His influence was as great in Quebec and British Columbia as it was in Ontario or elsewhere in Canada.

For those who had the privilege to be his students, the clarity, style and content of this book will come as no surprise. To others it will provide not only a source of new knowledge, but a perhaps unexpected reading pleasure.

Canadian Hospitals, 1920 to 1970 will undoubtedly be on the reading list of all schools of hospital administration. It carries a message for all categories of hospital workers; the trustee will gain a new understanding of his role, the hospital administrator will see the influence of sound and progressive administration on the growth of the hospital and improvement in care, the physician will gain an insight into the complexities of administration and the vital role the medical staff can play and must play in the betterment of hospital operation and the provision of total patient care.

Through this book, Harvey Agnew will continue to add to what was during his lifetime a most impressive contribution to the hospital field.

B.L.P. Brosseau, MD
Executive Director
Canadian Hospital Association

January 1973

Introduction

The publication of this book written by my revered friend and mentor of long standing, Harvey Agnew, is indeed a fitting tribute to a man who became known on the North American and indeed the world stage for his deep understanding and true appreciation of quality health services and, in particular, the important role played by hospitals within this setting.

Perhaps the most important aspect of Harvey's perception of hospitals was his keen insight of the fact that, while the clearest evidence of these institutions are the buildings of brick and mortar, their *real* significance in any community, and the contribution they can make to the well-being of mankind, is inextricably wrapped up in the attitudes, abilities and emphasis of all the people who make up the hospital family.

Harvey was, himself, an outstanding humanitarian.

I always considered myself extremely fortunate to have had the privilege of serving with Harvey from the time I first entered the field of hospital management. Those were the days when a few outstanding individuals, like Harvey, recognized the wide parameters of the art of true hospital management, which so greatly exceeded the basic business practices that frequently constituted the responsibilities of the superintendents or business managers of the time. To have had one's horizons lifted and broadened by his wise and sympathetic counselling was an experience which surely must parallel the deep satisfactions derived by the scholars who, centuries ago, sat at the feet of such unforgettable teachers as Plato, Aristotle, and Socrates.

That this book should be published after Harvey's passing is, again, quite understandable, as his primary efforts were continually directed toward personally passing along his ideas and concepts to younger people. He was ever-willing to share his store of knowledge with those of the succeeding generations, because it was through them he firmly believed would come a succession of more successful tomorrows.

Harvey Agnew's wide range of interests in life also made heavy demands on his time. But these, again, were some of the multiplicity of avenues which made frequent contacts with him such an enlightening experience. One quickly learned that while the immediacy of the health and hospital field was most important, life, to Harvey, also included a liberal sprinkling of many branches of the arts and sciences. To be his friend brought about as much mutual interest in these delights of living as did sharing companionship with him over good food and drink.

Canadian Hospitals, 1920 to 1970 will, therefore, forever reflect not only abundant fact, but, more important, perhaps, it will perpetuate the human touch which Harvey, through his amazing patience and warm feeling for people, managed to transfer so successfully to those of us who were fortunate enough to have him as a friend.

Stanley W. Martin, FCIS, FACHA
Deputy Minister of Health
Province of Ontario

February 1973

DEDICATED TO

Dr Malcolm T. MacEachern

whose indefatigable contributions to
hospital welfare and whose deep personal
interest in the welfare of others has
been an abiding inspiration;

AND TO MY WIFE

Mary Ann Johnson Agnew

who insisted that this historical record
be undertaken and who was of inestimable
help in its preparation.

Author's Introduction

The fifty-year period, 1920–70, was the most productive half century in the history of Canadian hospitals. More progress was made in those decades than in any previous comparable period. Since 1920 tremendous change has taken place in every aspect of hospital administration – in the distribution and provision of hospitals; in the development of a better quality of service through improved standards and regulations; in the better qualification of personnel at all levels; in medical, nursing and other types of education; in the scope of hospital activities; in greater government controls; in the development of hospital and medical insurance and other economic benefits; and in the efficiency of daily operation.

It is not the purpose of this study to review the individual history of the 1,400 hospitals in Canada; that would be a dull, even though historically rewarding, contribution to our archives. Rather, it is an effort to catalogue the progress which has been made over the half century and to examine the changes which have come about, some from within the hospital field and some as a result of broad changes beyond the field.

The fine hospitals of today are the result of the work of countless men and women who have made their contribution, small or large, to the advancement of our hospital knowledge, our facilities and our procedures. As well as the individual efforts, the inspired work of many associations must receive credit.

In this record, I will pay tribute to individuals, to those who led the way and made it possible for us to achieve today's successes. These persons were proud to make their own careers without endless assistance from others and devoted much of their time and substance to making life better for those less fortunate. One purpose of this volume is to record the names and efforts of many who served the cause of Canadian hospitals so faithfully over these years.[1]

It would not be fair, of course, to overlook the progress made in the last half of the nineteenth century. It was during this time that Lister developed antiseptic surgery and then aseptic surgery, procedures which quickly spread around the world and profoundly affected the nature and outcome of surgery in hospitals everywhere. The middle decades of this period also saw the identification of various pathogenic organisms by Pasteur, Rudolph Virchow, Koch, Behring and others; the isolation of these organisms was a long step towards the control of many diseases. Claude Bernard and a few of his contemporaries were making new discoveries in physiology. Nor should we overlook the concept of modern nursing, pioneered by England's Florence Nightingale and soon adopted in many countries. Canada's first school was the Mack School of Nursing established at the St Catharines General Hospital in 1874.

It *was* a half century of achievement. But the advances were mainly in medical knowledge. Except for the development of a new concept of nursing, comparatively little advance was made in hospital operation, in the scope of hospital care, in hospital financing or in hospital legislation.

The first twenty years of *this* century were characterized largely by advances in preventive medicine – the control of typhoid fever and of diphtheria – and of improvements in medical and nurse education. Hospitals everywhere installed X-ray equipment; usually the only available space was in the basement. Even smaller hospitals developed their own laboratories, also in basements, and we shudder now to think of some of the early techniques and interpretations. Most advances in that twenty-year period came from first world war activities. New techniques, such as *débridement*, were developed; new procedures, such as blood transfusions, became possible; and a number of outstanding military hospital administrators came back to become the civilian leaders of subsequent years.

---

1 At the time of his death Dr Agnew was reworking his manuscript to include his personal reminiscences of other leaders in the field of hospital administration. His notes indicate that he planned to write of numerous other friends and acquaintances including Dr J.J. Heagerty, Dr Helen MacMurchy, Mother Allaire, Dr Thomas W. Walker, Dr Gilbert Turner, Leonard Shaw, Rev John G. Fullerton, Father George Verrault, Percy Ward and many others. Because of the personal nature of Dr Agnew's perspective, the editors decided not to attempt to complete the task he had begun.

These and many other achievements of the previous decades comprise a fascinating story of evolution in the hospital field. But, significant though the achievements were, they were but the initial steps toward the momentum achieved in the half century reviewed in this book.

We are aware that everything is relative. In this study we compare what was available and accepted as 'modern' in the 1920s with what is now considered standard in the fine, present-day hospitals of the 1970s. We are proud of this progress and inwardly congratulate ourselves that we do not have to put up with the best they could muster in the twenties. Fifty years from now someone probably will be amused at our primitive equipment and futile attempts to cure various conditions. However, after another fifty years, someone may poke fun at the primitive concepts and techniques followed back in 2020 AD. There is some small consolation in that thought.

This book differs in one respect from many histories of a specific period. Frequently the personal observations of the writer, derived from a long contact with the scene, its changes and those who made them, are inserted into the narrative and elaborated. An economist or a long-time civil servant would write from quite a different viewpoint.

I have written this manuscript at the urging of many friends in the hospital field. It so happened that I was in close contact with hospitals across Canada during most of the period under consideration. In one capacity or another, I visited all but some of the more isolated hospitals, particularly in the late twenties and thirties. I knew nearly all of the administrators, then generally termed 'superintendents,' and a large percentage of the leading doctors. In recent years the ferryman on the River Styx has been very busy; it is a shock to realize that I am one of the few left who participated in a number of the early key developments during this period.

It is, therefore, with a sense of obligation to those who have gone before and with a sense of urgency that the annals of history shall be complete, that I look back, with considerable nostalgia, to the arduous but exciting and happy years that have gone.

G. Harvey Agnew, MD

Acknowledgements

While no one would be more anxious than Harvey Agnew to acknowledge everyone who gave him assistance in the writing of this book, it remains for those of us who were intimately involved in the organization of it after his untimely death, to thank those without whom he could not have confirmed the authenticity of his recollections. Therefore, if some of you have been omitted by name – and I know there must be many – the blame must be with me rather than with anyone else.

I regret that three men who gave much valuable advice did not live to see the finished book: Dr Angus McGugan, Edmonton; S.N. Wynn, Yorkton, Saskatchewan, and Dr W. Douglas Piercey, Halifax.

Besides these old friends, we remember Dr Duncan Graham, formerly Chief of Medicine, University of Toronto. Affectionately known as 'Old Dunc,' he was a guiding spirit not only when Harvey was a medical student, and, later, on the teaching staff, but the one who, while castigating him for leaving the field of internal medicine, still gave him encouragement and moral support when he entered the administrative field.

Many others gave great assistance both to the author and to those who had to polish off the manuscript. Among those were Dr J. C. Johnston, Calgary; Don Cox, Victoria, British Columbia; Dr L.O. Bradley, Canadian Council on Hospital Accreditation; Ruth Wilson, Moncton, New Brunswick; Dr C.J. Houston and S.H. Curran, Yorkton, Saskatchewan; Dr J.D. Griffith, Canadian Mental Health Association; Kenneth Ritchie, Department of Veterans Affairs; Dr James H. Graham, Royal College of Physicians and Surgeons; A.R. Shearer, Canadian Society of Laboratory

Technologists, as well as Ileen Kemp Parker, who started that organization; Dr W.S. Caldwell, Brampton, Ontario; Kenneth Muir, Brantford, Ontario; A.A. Mattila, Canadian Society of Radiological Technicians; Miss M.L. Parkin, Canadian Nurses Association; Dr C.U.L. Jeanes, Canadian Tuberculosis and Respiratory Disease Association; also, Dr Glen Sawyer, Ontario Medical Association, and Dr Arthur Kelly of both the Canadian and Ontario Medical Associations.

Two men, who not only gave us unstintingly of their time, but also put their staff members and records at our disposal, were Dr B.L.P. Brosseau, Executive Director, Canadian Hospital Association and Alan Hay, Executive Director, Ontario Hospital Association.

Eugenie Stuart, former professor in hospital administration, University of Toronto, gave valuable assistance with the chapter on nursing as did Joanne Waddington, Assistant Director, Atkinson School of Nursing, Toronto Western Hospital while Helen McArthur, Canadian Red Cross Society, contributed greatly with her observations and information about that organization.

There were many more. We hope that this volume will be of sufficient value to recompense them for the omission of their names.

Furthermore, we wish to thank the Ontario Hospital Association for its interest and financial support towards the research needed to compile this book and to Dr Agnew's consulting firm for the generous support in terms of office space, library facilities and other items.

Added to this, great credit must be given to Murray MacKenzie, Dr Agnew's research associate. Without him, the loose ends that remained after the sudden passing of Dr Agnew would never have been tied up – nor the manuscript completed as soon as it was. He did an outstanding job and I am greatly indebted to him. To this we must add a note of appreciation for the excellent job done by Mrs David Reed of Newmarket in the typing of the manuscript.

Finally, I personally wish to thank Ian Montagnes of the University of Toronto Press for his encouragement and fine editorial assistance in getting the manuscript ready for publication.

Only in completing a task such as this can one fully realize the many tried and true friends Harvey Agnew left behind.

Mary A. Agnew
Toronto, June 1973

CANADIAN HOSPITALS, 1920 TO 1970

1
Hospitals of the 1920s

Throughout colonial days and until the end of the nineteenth century, hospitals in Canada, as elsewhere, were little more than refuges for critically ill indigents and immigrants. Medicine had a limited basis in science and seriously ill patients were treated in the home whenever possible. Nursing care was given by friends and family according to the doctor's instructions. Hospitals were primarily charitable institutions for those who could not afford a private physician. It was not until the latter part of the nineteenth century that accommodations for private patients were built in Canadian hospitals.

In Canada, the earliest hospitals, many of which were established primarily for the treatment of Indians, were run under religious auspices. Writing of the pioneer Sisters who founded l'Hôtel-Dieu of Quebec in 1639 and l'Hôtel-Dieu of Montreal in 1642, the historian Francis Parkman noted that it would be difficult to conceive a self-abnegation more complete than that which they displayed in the course of their work and in their devotion to the sick:

In the almost total absence of trained and skilled physicians, the burden of (caring for) the sick and wounded fell upon them. Of the communities that of Montreal was the more wretchedly destitute, while that of Quebec was exposed, perhaps, to greater dangers. Nearly every ship from France brought some form of infection, and all infection found its way to the Hôtel-Dieu of Quebec. The nuns died but they never complained.[1]

1 Francis Parkman, *The Old Regime in Canada* (Boston: Little, Brown, 1874)

Besides these two hospitals and l'Hôpital Général of Quebec, five other hospitals were established during the French Regime. When the English assumed control of New France the struggling hospitals were cut off from their financial support in France and suffered accordingly. It was not until the 1840s that resources for new Catholic hospitals were accumulated. From that time until 1920 more than one hundred hospitals were built by such orders as the Grey Nuns, the Sisters of Providence, the Sisters of the Misericorde, the Sisters of St Joseph and many others. By no means restricting their activities to Quebec, these orders established charitable hospitals in the Maritimes and across the country. In many cases a close tie was maintained with the mother house of the order which set general policies and arranged for administration and staffing of its hospitals.

By the mid-nineteenth century a few hospitals had been built by secular groups motivated by a similar humanitarian concern for the sick poor. These voluntary groups formed non-profit hospital corporations. The memberships of the boards of trustees of these corporations varied considerably from city to city and from region to region but generally they included wealthy philanthropists and other influential community leaders interested in charitable works. The prime function of board members was to raise funds not only for the establishment and physical expansion of the hospital but also for continued maintenance. The local municipal government, or in rare cases the provincial government, occasionally appointed members to these boards of governors insofar as the governments contributed financially to the hospital. Some hospitals were municipally owned but the Victoria General Hospital in Halifax was the only provincially-owned general hospital before 1930.

Governments did build other types of hospitals such as asylums for the insane and isolation hospitals, although in Quebec these institutions were organized and operated by religious orders.

The voluntary hospital, whether lay or religious, was largely free from government control – only minimal standards had to be maintained by hospitals claiming subsidies for the care of indigents. In fact most hospitals operated in relative isolation one from the other. The first hospital associations were not established until the first decade of this century and even these faded into inactivity after a few years. The present hospital associations with their valuable educational programs date from the closing years of the second world war and later.

The conditions in nineteenth century hospitals were often desperate. Catholic hospitals often suffered from lack of funds. In the lay voluntary hospitals nurses were untrained and often indifferent to the needs of the patient. Although of higher moral standing than the undedicated, brandy-bibbling women of the Royal Hospitals, immortalized by Dickens as Sairey Gamps,[2] lay nurses were not respected and nursing in general was frowned upon as a vocation for any cultured woman.

In those days (1867) it was with the greatest difficulty patients could be induced to go into a hospital. It was the popular belief that if they went in they would never come out alive. No records were kept. The clinical thermometer had not come into use; the patients had to look after themselves; fresh air was not thought necessary. Armies of rats disported themselves about the wards. Instruments were looked after by a man who assisted in the operating room and at post mortems in the dead-house. Nothing was known of sepsis or antisepsis. Surgeons operated with dirty instruments and septic hands and wore coats which had been for years baptized with the blood of victims.[3]

Hospitals were scarce before 1870 and it was only during the 1870 to 1920 period with the rise of scientific medicine and the Nightingale system of nursing that the hospital came to be generally accepted as a superior institution for medical care. This public acceptance took many years, however, and was by no means complete by 1920. Furthermore, some patients avoided hospitals because of their exorbitant costs – about $1.50 per day for the public wards and up to $3.00 per day for a private room in the years immediately after the first world war. By and large, however, as people became increasingly prosperous, they grew more willing to be hospitalized when necessary. This increased public acceptance encouraged the growth of more and better institutional facilities.

The precise number of hospitals and of hospital beds in 1920 is not known. In addition, other statistics related to the extent and distribution of hospitals and particular hospital services or functions were either not computed, unreliable or misplaced over the years.

In 1930, Dr Helen MacMurchy, Director of the Division of Child Welfare

2 The 'Sairey Gamps' were the nurses who manned the Royal Hospitals after Henry VIII closed the monastic hospitals about 1530. As the hospitals were continued under lay direction there followed a very dark page in nursing history. Sir Henry Burdett stated in *The History of the London Hospital* that 'every vice was rampant among those women whose only aid to the dying was to remove pillows and bed clothes and so hasten the end.' They were adept, too, at removing jewellery and anything else of value.

3 Dr F.J. Shepherd, a leading Montreal physician, speaking to the Montreal General Hospital Nurses Club, 1905, quoted in J.J. Heagerty, *Four Centuries of Medical History in Canada* (Toronto: Macmillan, 1928), vol.2. p. 144

in the Department of Pensions and National Health and then in charge of the federal program to reduce maternal mortality (still extensive in the days before antibiotics) realized the need for better hospital statistics. She proposed to me that the federal government would publish a directory of hospitals if the Canadian Medical Association's Department of Hospital Service, of which I was then secretary, would undertake to compile the data. The department agreed to the arrangement but we found it difficult to get an accurate picture of existing facilities in some provinces, much less an indication of what had existed in the past. Only three or four of the provinces had good data and none had space requirement standards for each bed, so that submitted figures were of set up complement rather than 'rated' capacity. If space requirements had been applied then as in later years the bed total reported would have been significantly lower.

In 1929 figures for hospitals and beds were:

Type	Hospitals	Beds
Public general[4] (including general paediatric and Red Cross)	481	32,218
Tuberculosis institutions	31	5,655
General paediatric hospitals	14	909
Orthopaedic hospitals	12	512
Public maternity hospitals	25	1,719
Total maternity accommodation (estimated)		6,000+
Department of Pensions and National Health	16	3,614
Mental and neurological hospitals	42	26,862
Red Cross hospitals, outposts and nursing stations	47	401
Private hospitals	269	2,500 (approx.)
Hospitals for incurables	33	2,700 (approx.)
Convalescent hospitals	9	325
Total	886	74,882

4 U.S. readers may find it confusing that certain widely-used terms have differing meanings in the two countries. In the United States a 'public' hospital is one which is owned and supported by the community, e.g., Bellevue in New York City and Cook County Hospital in Chicago. In Canada a 'public' hospital has traditionally been one which is non-profit and has received financial help from the province, originally for the care of indigents; the hospital may be municipally owned or (and this is the difference) may be a voluntary one, e.g., a Sisters' hospital or the Winnipeg General or the Royal Jubilee in Victoria. What

Because certain tuberculosis, orthopaedic, paediatric, mental and maternity hospitals were listed under more than one category the total in the figures above is not a direct summation of each type of hospital. In addition, some of the institutions listed would not be considered hospitals by more recent and stringent standards. For example, many of the institutions claiming to be private hospitals provided little more than room and board with virtually no medical supervision.

More reliable statistics for 1933, at which time there were about 45,000 beds in 589 public hospitals,[5] show that there were 486 hospitals with departments of radiology, 299 with clinical laboratories, 230 with physical therapy departments and 119 with out-patient departments.

Then, as now, some provinces and regions were much better endowed than others. Urban industrialized areas have always supported most of the large, complex and specialized active treatment institutions. Despite the tremendous outpost hospital efforts of the Red Cross and other religious and charitable organizations, health services in many northern regions of the country were minimal or non-existent. For example there were only six small hospitals in the Northwest Territories and the Yukon and these were staffed permanently by graduate nurses and their assistants only during the 1920s.

Although there were shortages of most types of hospital beds, the severest gaps in hospital care concerned the inadequacy of treatment and facilities for the mentally ill, extended-care patients and the tuberculous.

Conditions in Hospitals
The almost unbelievable conditions within hospitals during the mid-nineteenth century had been long since corrected by 1920, except perhaps for the lack of clinical records in some less progressive hospitals. However, the hospital itself was a far cry from those of today.

The larger hospitals were basically horizontal in design rather than vertical and tended to be of the pavillion type. They were characterized by large public wards, a never-adequate number of semi-private rooms and an equally insufficient number of single rooms. In smaller towns in the east the hospital was often a converted large home, donated by the family of

---

Canadians call a voluntary hospital, the Americans often refer to as 'private' although there is an increasing use of the term 'voluntary.' A 'private' hospital – that is, one operated for profit (if any) by a private individual or group – is called 'proprietary' in the United States.
5 Not including mental hospitals.

a pioneer lumberman or local merchant. Patients would be scattered all through the building including a few in the domestic's quarters on the third floor. When the hospitals had been converted from private homes the corridors, stairs and bedroom doors were often too narrow, plumbing was inadequate and the staff spent most of its time toiling up and down the stairs. Frequently, when a more modern addition would be added, the old original part was still preserved, perpetuating much of the inefficiency of layout and facilities.

The public wards ranged in capacity from eight to ten beds in smaller hospitals to thirty to thirty-six and more in large hospitals. They were low in privacy and noise control, but rated well in other respects. They were spacious, remarkably well ventilated, usually cheerful and the days seemed much shorter than in private rooms. There was always something of interest happening. It was comforting to have nurses always in sight day or night and there was always some up-patient ready to bring a glass of water or pick up something from the floor. While there was more noise and disturbance at times, these were usually less annoying in the big rooms than the noises and chatter and smoke of the two- or three-bed rooms. Bed curtains on rods or tracks had not yet been invented and one major disturbance when windows were open was the sudden overturning of the portable bed screens. Their wooden frames made a tremendous clatter, particularly at night. Another annoyance was the almost constant smell of burning rubber; nurses would boil catheter or bottle nipples in enamel saucepans and let them boil dry while they rushed off to other duties. The stench of burning rubber throughout the floor set nurses running as fast as their ankle-length skirts would permit to remove the offending mess. We were resigned to air pollution in those days.

The few private rooms were usually small. Few had either washbasins or waterclosets. The corridor bedpan parade to the soiled-utility room was a normal ritual. By the late 1920s the floor- or wall-type bedpan washes were replacing the hopper. Larger hospitals had a few VIP rooms with a watercloset and sometimes a tub. If present, the latter was seldom used and often decked with a wooden cover on which spare linen or the patient's suitcases were stored. Showers were practically non-existent. When it became obvious that the private room should have a toilet, in keeping with the trend in first-class hotels, the facilities were frequently shared by two adjoining rooms, an arrangement which resulted in much bad language and the scurrying of nurses to unhook, or unbolt, the door from the other side. Room phones did not exist except when especially installed for some more-or-less permanent patient. Some rooms had outlets so that a phone could be plugged in if requested. Some hospitals had a pay phone mounted on a dolly connected by a very long cord to its base down the corridor. This could be wheeled in on request.

It was the height of sophisticated hospital design at that time to hide pipes in the wall so as not to offend the eye. It was not considered necessary to put in access panels and the pipes were often buried in concrete. Copper piping was almost never used. No one seemed to think of the future. It was unfortunate, too, that this practice came in a period when buildings were constructed to last forever. Untold thousands of dollars have been spent by hospital boards trying to find and then replace worn out and leaking pipes.

Most bedrooms had an all-purpose centre ceiling light – hardly conducive to reading in bed. Gooseneck and clamp-on reading lights were improvised. Movable floor lamps were being tried out in a few hospitals. The useful removable gatch frame under the mattress was coming into use but was not built as part of the bed and satisfactorily motorized until the late 1930s. There were no overbed tables as yet. Manufacturers were beginning to experiment with more useful bedside tables. Window sills were invariably placed so high that a patient in a chair could see only tree tops and clouds.

There was practically no automation as we understand it. A few procedures in radiology, in the boiler plant, in the kitchen and in the laundry were automatically controlled, but the concept was not generally applied. Automatic controls on elevators were just being introduced; most were staff operated. In many smaller hospitals the elevator was still operated by pulling a rope inside the cab. There were no automatic dishwashers, laundry washers, central dispatch equipment, auto-analyzers, or automatically recorded sterlizing controls.

Operating lighting was incandescent, simple in structure and produced excessive heat for the operating staff. A favorite form was a large suspended pipe ring with as many as ten or more single lights arranged around it. It did reduce shadows to a degree. Many emergency rooms had nothing more than a large light surmounted by a white enamel reflector. The first 'shadowless' light, the Scialytic, was just becoming popular in France and experimentally tested in Canada. Towards the end of this decade considerable interest was being created by the Holophane method of lighting, a system of glass squares arranged in a large ceiling panel which were designed to refract the rays from the individual lights behind them so that they concentrated on the operative site. By controlling them as separate banks, light could be directed down at different angles of incidence.

Electrical wiring was usually inadequate. The use of electrical appliances was multiplying, and as a result of their limited number each outlet looked like a bedraggled Medusa. Blown fuses at the most inopportune moment were just part of hospital life; the overheating of wires through the use of over-capacity fuses, not to mention coins, must have resulted in gray hairs for many hospital engineers.

Few hospitals had adequate emergency current. Some had battery operated corridor and operating room pedestal lights. Some rural hospitals wisely kept a few Coleman gasoline lamps in reserve. Few, if any, had emergency power for elevators or pumps or, later, oil-fired boilers. It was not until the power shortages caused by accelerated industrial activity during the first world war hit some of the more thickly populated areas and left hospitals for hours with little or no power, that hospitals installed emergency power systems. Some of these, diesel or gas, were exceedingly efficient, and in some instances fully duplicated the normal power requirements.

It is of interest that Ontario, which had pioneered the development of inexpensive hydro-electric power on this continent, was not reaping the full advantage of its program because of the unfortunate choice of twenty-five cycle rather than sixty cycle production. Until the province-wide changeover to sixty cycle took place in the late forties, the hospitals in Ontario had to pay a premium on their scientific electrical equipment because of the special wiring required. Later, if the equipment was sold it had to be sold to another Ontario hospital or the potential market was reduced to users of sixty-cycle current. A few of the hospitals in the 1920s still used direct current, either purchased locally or produced by their own equipment. This was probably advantageous at the time but required changeover to permit use of the modern equipment in constant use in hospitals.

There was no vinyl flooring, so easy to maintain. For corridors the favorite flooring was battleship linoleum, terrazzo or cork; for bedrooms, hardwood tongue-and-groove, battleship linoleum or terrazzo; for operating and delivery rooms, terrazzo or ceramic tile; for kitchens, quarry tile; for offices and dining rooms, hardwood tongue-and-groove; for laboratories, radiology and emergency rooms, battleship linoleum.

The kitchen was almost invariably too small; all too often it was the kitchen of the original building now serving a bed complement three or four times greater than planned for. Many hospitals still cooked with coal, a few in isolated northern areas with wood and, in cities, frequently with the manufactured gas used in homes. Natural gas was unknown except in oil- and gas-producing areas. Dishwashers were few in number and comparatively primitive; pot washers came much later. Electrical cooking was expensive and only a few used it to any extent. When I began to visit hospitals methodically in the late twenties the arch enemy of many kitchen staffs was the host of mice, cockroaches and silverfish.

Heating was largely by coal except in some of the oil- and gas-producing areas. Well into the forties many hospital engineers were convinced that coal was both less costly and more reliable than oil; I recall frequent discussions on this topic. Natural gas was still to be piped to many regions and electric heating was still a long time in the future. During the depression and later, a number of British Columbia hospitals experimented with sawdust as a fuel available there in large quantities. However, it required extensive storage space and stoking was a labor and mechanical problem.

The biggest problem with coal, apart from the ubiquitous dust, was the frequent breakdown of the worm mechanism feeding coal to the boiler. The spiral worms would be sheared off by bolts, horseshoes, and other metal articles in the coal.

The prevailing heating system was forced hot water, complete with intermittent banging where the single pipe circuit was used. Steam gave quicker heat but usually kept the nurses running to turn it on or off; it was all 'roast or freeze.' The vacuum steam system was better but seemed to require much central adjustment. Forced hot air was then considered too dusty and unhygienic. (The refinements in this system which now make it so popular were yet to come.) Radiant heating was being developed in Europe but at that time was still untried in Canadian hospitals. Smoke pollution was a serious problem but was accepted as part of life.

Ventilation was almost entirely by natural means, which meant open, albeit, screened windows. One of the early morning tasks was to wipe the fine coal dust off the window sills; I often watched this procedure in the operating and delivery rooms. Efforts at humidification were rather primitive and comparatively ineffectual except where steam heating was used and a steam radiator would be tapped.

The hazard of fire was much greater a half century ago than it is now. Today, provincial requirements both for initial construction and for daily operation are so stringent that many architects and administrators feel that they are unnecessarily restrictive, particularly in view of the constant twenty-four hour usage of almost all parts of the hospital. Nevertheless, there have been some tragic hospital fires and it is prudent to play safe in spite of the considerable addition to costs.

Fifty years ago restrictions on fire-resistant buildings of steel or concrete frame seemed adequate enough but were far from present-day requirements. Elevator shafts were open as were stairways. Corridors were not sealed by self-closing doors unless (in some provinces) leading to a wing built of wood. Tanks of oxygen and other gases were often stored in a room without an outside window. The cautery, to my personal knowledge, was often used in the presence of ether. Shortly after the Cleveland clinic holocaust I witnessed a radiologist thoughtlessly lay a glowing cigarette on a pile of the old, highly inflammable cellulose nitrate X-ray film. The duties of nurses and other staff in case of fire were usually posted. But with frequent transfers from one floor to another or from one duty to another, the individual was often confused at the time of fire drill. In the course of my visits I found many extinguishers with plugged nozzles or otherwise unusable. Some neatly hung firehoses had not been off the hooks in years; a number were rotted. Some wooden buildings were being 'sprinklered' and thermo-detectors were gradually being installed in unused portions of old buildings. Over the years local and provincial fire marshals and their inspectors have done a great deal to remove the fire hazard from hospitals. The medical profession, too, has done much to make it safer for the patients.

The small operating pit surrounded by a steep bank of seats for large numbers of students, immortalized in various paintings of famous clinicians, were rare in Canadian teaching hospitals after the first world war. There were quite a number, however, still in use in the United States, in Britain and on the continent. They did provide a comparatively vertical view for the student, although those at the back must have seen very little and the steps down were precipitous. One shudders to think of the clouds of bacteria that must have settled down on the operating field and the impossibility of separating completely sterile and unsterile areas in such a small confined space.

My most vivid impression of this type of teaching theatre was of that at the Lankeneau Hospital in Philadelphia, which was typical. My chief in New York, where I was interning, had told me that my education would be deficient if I did not spend a few days listening to and observing the techniques of John B. Deaver, the internationally famous surgeon at Lankenau.

I travelled to Philadelphia and on the first morning I sat high up in the back row. Although the attendance was large, Dr Deaver must have known his regulars well for he gave the stranger a sharp look several times during the operation. When it was over he called me down to the rim of the pit.

'You're a visitor?'

'Yes, I am.'

'Welcome. What's your name and where are you from?'

I told him.

'Any relation to D. Hayes?'

I knew what he meant. Dr D. Hayes Agnew was considered the greatest of the surgeons of the seaboard states from the time of the Civil War, in which he served conspicuously, through the decades to his death in 1892. He was professor of surgery at the University of Pennsylvania, a great teacher and author and was brought in as consultant when President James A. Garfield was fatally shot in Washington. I replied that Dr D. Hayes Agnew and my family had come from the same part of Ireland but, as far as I knew, we were not related.

John B. Deaver was stripping off his rubber gloves and his hands were white with talcum powder. He reached up and laid a dusty hand on my sleeve.

'My boy, whenever you are anywhere in this area, always claim D. Hayes Agnew as an uncle.'

FIFTY YEARS OF TRANSITION

Changes and improvements have a tendency to slip up on us so gradually that we often absorb them into our life, or let them materially change the direction of our lives, without consciously realizing what transformations are happening. In the hospital field many minor alterations occur every year, yet it is only when we look back a few decades that we realize what a sum total of changes has taken place.

To look back fifty years does bring the transition and its contrasts into sharp focus. While the individual hospital may have been ahead of its time in some details and could indignantly dissociate itself from the list below, I believe the list fairly depicts the picture of the day as it related to the vast majority of the general hospitals of the early 1920s.

1 *General patient care*

No intensive care units.

No coronary care units.

No post-anaesthetic room (few hours only).

No recovery room in surgery (twenty-four-hour coverage).

No recovery or observation room in delivery.

No holding or observation room in emergency.

No blood transfusion service. The better hospitals used citrated blood, or transfused by the multiple syringe technique, a tricky procedure. Some used the Unger or other mechanical equipment to improve the syringe technique. Blood grouping was not reliable. The valuable Red Cross blood service did not come into being until after the first world war. Blood banks were non-existent.

No prepared glucose, sterile saline or other intravenous preparations. Some hospitals had elaborate setups to make their own sterile solutions.

No sulfa drugs.

No penicillin and other antibiotic drugs.

Insulin was just being made available to a few hospitals on an experimental basis.

Vitamins were just being differentiated and their functions becoming clarified.

Hormone treatments were being introduced but there was still much confusion about inter-glandular relationships.

No anti-coagulants such as heparin or dicumerol.

No bone banks.

No eye banks.

No Salk vaccine for poliomyelitis.

No disposables, as we use the term today.

No central sterilizing and supply department.

No radios (except an occasional 'peanut tube' set).

No television for patients.

No iodized salt. (Considerable hyperthyroidism prevailed, particularly in the Great Lakes area.)

Morphia and other narcotics were kept on open shelves in the pharmacy and almost as carelessly on the nursing floors.

Few sterile vial injections preparations.

Many drugs in tablet form had to be boiled with water over the 'hypodermic lamp' and individual arithmetic calculations made for the dosage to be given.

2 *Medical procedures*

Most anaesthetic induction was by ethyl chloride spray from a hand-held glass tube, followed by ether dropped on a mask from a can with a small cotton wick attached. Sometimes nitrous oxide was used, either to induct or for short operations. Some of the 'old timers' still used straight chloroform or an ACE mixture (alcohol, chloroform and ether). Except in teaching or other large hospitals, most of the anaesthetics were given by the referring doctor (unless he preferred to assist the surgeon), or by a member of the staff giving anaesthetics as a complement to his general practice.

No organ transplants.

No cardio-pulmonary investigation.

There was considerable controversy as to whether the portable machines for doing the basal metabolic rate were as accurate as the large bench type van Slyke apparatus. The protein-bound iodine test (PB 1) for detecting hyperthyroidism had not yet been developed.

No cobalt-90 or cesium equipment; high dosage radiation was still in the research stage.

No isotopes for diagnosis or treatment.

No angiography, cardiac catheterization or mammography.

Radium in plaques or needles was still a favorite treatment for malignancy.[6]

Electrocardiograph equipment, compact enough to be portable, was coming on the market but was still only available in the larger hospitals and in a few private offices. The extensive range of electronic equipment was still in the future.

In radiology there was no ciné equipment and no video. Automatic developing did not come for many years. The fire-hazardous cellulose nitrate radiological films were generally used. Only after the holocaust at the Crile Clinic in Cleveland, May 15, 1929, did the use of the slow-burning and much safer cellulose acetate film become generally used and mandatory in most provinces and states. Although film had been used exclusively for some years, a surprisingly large number of hospital personnel still referred to them as 'plates.'

In the laboratory microchemical procedures were just being developed by Killian and others. Auto-analyzers, flame photometers, cell counters, et cetera, were unknown. The first time-saving device introduced in this period was the auto-technicon for staining slides.

3 *Other hospital facilities and services*

No two-way voice nurse-call system. Usually there was only a push-button on a cord and a light over the door.

No centralized dietary service except in quite small short-carry hospitals. The staff cafeteria was elementary.

No automatic consoles for dispensing cigarettes, soft drinks, et cetera.

No electric refrigerators. Ice boxes were still in use. Many smaller hospitals still had their own ice house, complete with sawdust and a rinsing hose.

No computer service (until the sixties).

No machine accounting; no electric typewriters.

No radio paging for doctors and key staff.

A few hospitals had women's auxiliaries but display and sales shops in the lobby did not develop to any extent until the thirties. Most of the early cigarette and magazine booths set up, often in the basement near the dining room, were operated by trainees of the Canadian National Institute for the Blind.

This is an amazing list of what hospitals did *not* have in the 1920s. It

---

6 The Radium Institute in Toronto, founded many years earlier by Dr W.H.B. Aikins, was carried on through the 1920s by Dr F. Arnold Clarkson and Dr Fred M. Harrison. It dealt only with radium treatments.

could readily be lengthened if we were to review the many facilities which we have now in general hospitals.

In the light of what hospitals did not provide in the twenties one could readily believe that hospital care must have been inadequate and seriously limited. At the time it did not seem so. We did not realize what we did not know. We were tremendously impressed with the advances we were making, such as the discovery of insulin by Banting, Best and their colleagues; Minot's conquest of pernicious anaemia (although an extract of liver was not yet developed and patients had to eat liver in countless forms to vary the monotony of the diet); advances in blood transfusion knowledge and techniques; delivery by version; *débridement*; plastic surgery, and other procedures coming out of the first world war. Lung surgery and early segregation were clearing up tuberculosis more rapidly than open terraces in winter.

Many diseases were still baffling. Poliomyelitis was still a recurring scourge; tuberculosis still took its toll albeit a lessening one; rheumatic fever and its sequelae were all too prevalent and treatment was largely palliative. The doctors of the day were masters of their craft, dedicated to their work and many were outstanding teachers. Moreover they had fewer distractions than their modern counterparts and developed a concentration which would be difficult to achieve now.

Nurses of the day had never heard of electronic monitoring, nor of electrolytic imbalance, but they were intelligent, devoted to their work, loyal and not particularly concerned with more time off, overtime pay, fringe benefits and other matters of so much concern today. If patients still needed nursing care after seven o'clock, the nurses stayed on without further thought. In the thirties some of the urban hospitals adopted the eight-hour schedule, but it replaced the twelve-hour arrangement rather slowly in many hospitals.

While the teaching hospitals and a number of the larger non-teaching hospitals had a limited number of interns, the great majority of hospitals did not have any such help. Certification in specialties was yet to come and most residencies, after one year of general internship (occasionally two), were in general surgery, general medicine, obstetrics and gynaecology, paediatrics and a few, only, of the subspecialties, particularly otolaryngology and ophthalmology. The number of residents was limited compared with today's legions.

Of necessity, the attending doctors had to keep in close daily contact with their public- (now standard-) ward patients. Many minor procedures ordered had to be done by the physicians themselves, for nurses were not permitted to undertake as many of these tasks as they do now. For example, blood pressure readings and intramuscular injections were not generally done by nurses. The removal of stitches was a ceremonial procedure performed only by a doctor, usually the operating surgeon himself.

What would at present be viewed as a lamentable dearth of plumbing on patients' floors resulted in a constant parade throughout the day, particularly of nurses with bedpans and wash water, or of patients being helped to the washrooms. Catheters, duodenal tubes, finger cots and other rubber articles were usually boiled on the utility room gas plate or electric plate (no central sterilizing then).

SOME PERSONAL REMINISCENCES

Many episodes crowd the mind as I think back to my early years in medicine.

Early in the first world war and after I had completed my third year of the five-year medical course I spent my vacation as a 'summer intern' at the (then) forty-bed Ross Memorial Hospital at Lindsay, Ontario. It seemed to be a good opportunity of gaining some hospital experience, but I do not think the matron of the hospital realized how little I knew about clinical medicine. I learned a lot about smaller hospitals that summer; on the whole, it was typical of rural hospitals of the period.

Any one of the medical staff could do his own surgery but some were not interested and others did only what they could do safely. Most of the surgery was done by two doctors. Each of the others administered his own anaesthetics; a nurse (or that summer, I) served as the assistant. No one gave nitrous oxide, the usual induction being with ethyl chloride spray (or chloroform, in some instances) followed by straight ether and a short-lived wrestling match. There was no medical orgaization to my knowledge, although one of the surgeons was generally considered to be chief of staff. Four of the doctors drove model T's or the equivalent, but the others clung to their horse and carriage. The chairman of the board, J.D. Flavelle, brother of Sir Joseph Flavelle, was a conscientious citizen and devoted Sunday afternoons to the hospital. As he was of Falstaffian proportions, the matron, a nurse of the old school and herself a generous silhouette, gave me stern instructions to be sure that the strongest chair in the hospital would be in her office on Sundays for Mr Flavelle's visit. We – the nurses and I – dubbed it 'the throne.'

That summer's 'most unforgettable character' was the senior surgeon, Dr J.A.D. McAlpine. A brother-in-law of Sir Sam Hughes, the minister of defence, Dr McAlpine had much of the same spirit of independence and utter disregard for 'red tape,' protocol and conventional procedure. He had theories on a wide range of subjects, but particularly on physiology. He spent hours giving his views on physiology and reiterating that most of the teaching at the university was wrong. I was never able to judge whether he was right or wrong for our professor of physiology mumbled to himself hour after hour. He never got anything across to the students except that all other physiologists were wrong. We could set our watches by his actions, however. At four minutes to the hour he got out a cigarette; at two minutes to the hour he got out a wooden match; with thirty seconds to go the cigarette went to his mouth and the mumbling became even less audible. With eyes on the clock, he waited until the second hand was vertical, then with a deft movement the match was ignited on the table, applied to the cigarette and he was slowly on his way. What we learned we got from Halliburton's textbook.

Dr McAlpine did not wear rubber gloves when operating – he never had and never would. In spite of this idiosyncracy, his record was good for he appears to have had no more post-operative infections or stitch abscesses than the others. Unfortunately, the almost complete absence of worthwhile clinical records made it impossible to check his broad observation. More than once I saw perspiration drop from his face into the abdomen. At other times I saw him push his spectacles back on his nose with his bare hand and then go back to searching for an elusive appendix or gall bladder. His claim was that the peritoneum can handle a few organisms without difficulty; it is only extensive contaminations that overwhelm the defensive powers of the body.

On one occasion the surgery planned required an outside surgeon. Dr Herbert A. Bruce, chief surgeon of the Wellesley Hospital in Toronto and later Lieutenant-Governor of Ontario, was summoned. He arrived on the morning train, confirmed the diagnosis and arranged for the operation. Dr McAlpine was to assist. Then the altercation began. Dr Bruce insisted that Dr McAlpine wear gloves; the older man objected. They argued interminably to my unbounded delight, but finally Dr McAlpine gave in.

In those days rubber gloves were not dusted with powder and slipped on dry; they were usually boiled, filled with sterile water and the hand was 'floated' in. It was a difficult technique, especially in getting the fingers inserted to the tips. Dr McAlpine was neither experienced in the procedure nor was he in the mood to co-operate. He shredded the cuffs on a month's supply of gloves before Dr Bruce was satisfied that his assistant's gloves were sufficiently on to permit him to use his fingers.

Intern life in the twenties was considerably different from what it became in subsequent decades. During the war years interns were almost impossible to find. Senior students took over the interns' duties as best they could. Students and interns disappeared overnight into the services and new faces appeared – usually students sent home to finish their courses before returning overseas as graduates.

The civilian hospitals felt the first world war severely. Doctors, nurses and other personnel enlisted in considerable numbers and staff work suffered. Those who remained, particularly the medical staff, had to assume added responsibilities. In teaching hospitals the shortages were noticeable. A number of the larger teaching hospitals, in co-operation with their affiliated medical schools, set up and staffed base or other military hospitals with the officers and key personnel almost entirely drawn from the civilian hospital group. Examples would be the teaching hospitals of McGill, Toronto, Laval, and Queen's, which set up four of the sixteen general hospitals mobilized overseas.

This situation made it not only difficult to maintain the normal work of the teaching hospitals but was a hardship on the medical students whose teaching was undertaken or completed by junior staff men, often new appointees. Impelled by patriotism and a desire to be actively engaged in the war effort, medical students enlisted in great numbers, despite contrary advice from the Royal Canadian Army Medical Corps (RCAMC) and school authorities. Most of these students were returned to their studies; some went back to war as doctors, not combatants.

The shortages of medical staff, of nurses and of technical personnel were extremely serious. The hospitals competed with war industry and other occupations for less-skilled personnel. Equipment of all kinds was in short supply because of diversion overseas. Construction was exceedingly limited if not impossible because of the limited amount of steel and other materials available for civilian use.

Following the war the civilian hospitals and, of course, the public gained in two ways. First, the returning doctors, nurses and technicians brought back new techniques and concepts which advanced the quality of services. Second, a number of doctors who had served overseas had become interested in administrative work; some chose not to go back to clinical work. A number of them went into the administrative field and became, instead, administrative heads of some of our leading hospitals. Instances coming to mind are Dr S.R.D. Hewitt of the Regina General Hospital and later the Saint John General Hospital; Dr R.T. Washburn of the University Hospital in Edmonton; and Dr Fred C. Bell of the Vancouver General Hospital and later of Shaughnessy Veterans' Hospital. (In addition to his devoted hospital work on the West Coast, 'Freddie' Bell was also a dedicated mountain climber. He served as president of the Alpine Club of Canada for a time and in later years was its librarian. He died in 1971 at the age of 89.)

During 1919 and 1920, the period of demobilization, many recent graduates (and many experienced doctors, too) sought additional hospital training before establishing their practice. Many of the general practitioners leaving the armed forces decided to specialize and the hospital directors of various specialty services received enquiries as never before. For once there was a surplus of graduates and the large hospitals could pick and choose.

The senior year arrangements across Canada varied. Some of the universities such as McGill, Western Ontario and Manitoba, made the final year an academic one; the internship came after graduation and was served where the graduate desired. Others such as Toronto, Queen's, Montreal and Dalhousie included a one-year internship as the final year, usually with some academic work included; these schools specified the hospitals in which the graduate should intern, usually a hospital close by the graduating institution.

In my own case, I served as a junior intern at the Toronto Western Hospital in my final year. For most of that time there were no senior interns or residents – all able-bodied graduates were in the services. Along with our regular duties in the wards, surgery, emergency and so on, we junior interns had to spend a certain number of hours each week in military training. Our 'free time' was non-existent. To add to the problems in that confused period, teachers and staff doctors were coming and going, as the high command of the RCAMC shifted personnel to keep the medical schools operating.

Later, after graduation, I had planned to return to Great Britain where the chief surgeon of a large teaching hospital had offered me a minor position. I arrived in New York during a dock strike and all sailings were cancelled indefinitely. After waiting a month with no strike settlement in sight, I obtained a temporary position on the intern staff of the Harlem Division of the Bellevue and Allied Hospital system. This hospital, with its excellent attending staff, had a reputation for the most exciting emergency service in the city. In addition, its obstetrical service was said to have more abnormalities than any other. My subsequent experience bore this out. In the years since my internship in Bellevue's Harlem branch, the hospital and its administration have become involved in the New York political situation and, regrettably, appointments there are not sought as they were then. Dr Norman M. Guiou, gynaecologist for many years at the Ottawa Civic Hospital and now retired, was a close associate during that period.

Competition for internship posts in the u.s., as in Canada, was fierce. My position (a temporary one at first) was coming up for competition by examination. When it was announced that 129 candidates were going to write, I got down to work as never before. I wrote case histories before the staff arrived; I performed tests and did laboratory work before they were ordered. The chief had never had such service. A few hours before the examination, the chief of service advised me not to worry – he had made his decision. Just the same I wrote the examination carefully, in case I had misunderstood his meaning. A week later he officially welcomed me on staff.

Internship then was less rigidly controlled than is the case now. There was no CMA approval of hospitals for internship (the approval plan was implemented in 1931). There was no Canadian Association of Medical Students and Interns (CAMSI) to work out a matching arrangement for applicants and available positions. Graduate internships were at that time a matter of agreement between the graduate and the hospital. There was usually an intern committee on the staff but few hospitals had a medical director, as such, or an assistant superintendent (medical) to direct the work of the interns. Most graduates took one year of internship, a few took two.

After my internship in New York, I returned to Toronto and was eventually placed in charge of female medicine at the Toronto Western Hospital under the direction of Dr F. Arnold Clarkson, the physician-in-chief. One of my interns during this period of the twenties was Dr Robert McClure who was later to become well known as a medical missionary and as the first lay moderator of the United Church of Canada. When he worked as one of my interns, Bob McClure was a bundle of boundless energy but he could seldom be found when needed on the ward. When I realized that he spent every minute available following emergency and surgical procedures in preparation for his mission hospital career, I had no heart to chide him for ward absenteeism.

There were only a few residents in the twenties and they worked mainly in the major teaching hospitals. There was no prescribed course nor length of time to be served – the Royal College of Physicians and Surgeons of Canada had not yet been established with its prescribed years of postgraduate training and examinations to qualify for certification. Nor had the well known 'Gallie' course in surgery been set up by Dr E.W. Gallie, of the University of Toronto, the first full-length qualification course for a major specialty in this country. Specialty boards were being set up in the United States but it was not until the 1930s that a correlating committee was set up to approve specialty boards and to delay approval of others until certain weaknesses were overcome. I sat on this joint board in its early years as a representative of the American Hospital Association, along with Dr Robin C. Buerki, one of the AHA's outstanding leaders.

In that period, as for many preceding decades, it was a common practice for young Canadian graduates to go to Great Britain to take their 'fellowship' (FRCS) either in London or in Edinburgh. Others qualified for their MRCP. French-speaking graduates took their postgraduate work in Paris. The training in Great Britain heavily stressed the basic sciences of anatomy and physiology rather than the technical skills of operative surgery. In this respect the FRCS examinations differed from those of the American College of Surgeons in which emphasis was laid upon operative experience and ability; extensive case reports were required as part of the submission to the ACS.

Vienna was still a mecca for many graduates. It had the advantage of a wide variety of courses in English or German, courses that extended from a few weeks to many months. These courses could be entered at any time as part of a group or as an individual. Assistantships to good surgeons could be obtained in various hospitals in Austria or in Hungary for approximately a hundred dollars per month. Vienna became a leader in medicine when the Empress Maria Theresa decreed in the eighteenth century that all patients dying in the public hospitals could be subjected to post-mortem examination. This gave Vienna a tremendous early lead in pathology, the basis of medical knowledge. In more recent years the costly nature of present-day research has made it exceedingly difficult for a small country like Austria to sponsor elaborate medical research efforts.

Internships were unpaid positions in the twenties, and so were most of the residencies. Interns and residents alike 'earned' their meals, rooms and uniforms only. Living out was unknown among the interns and not a common practice among the residents. Few interns were married and neither were many of the residents. Most residents served only one or two years following their internship. A fair number of medical school graduates, on completion of their internship went to the United States for specialized training. One factor was the desire for a broader learning experience; another was the possibility of a paying position. Interns in the U.S. were seldom paid by the well-known hospitals but a salary was offered by a few, mainly non-teaching hospitals in smaller cities as a means of attracting graduates.

(Today's interns and residents do much better than their counterparts of the twenties. In the early seventies, an intern in Canadian hospitals may expect to be paid between $5,000 and $7,000 a year. Residents may draw between $8,000 and $13,000 a year. One can readily understand why many medical schools are replacing their requirements for internship with final-year, medical clerkships.)

The interns of the twenties worked to a timetable – a strenous one – but the clock meant little when there were patients to be treated. My own experience was typical.

We worked six and one-half days a week and had every second Sunday afternoon off. During the week we had alternate evenings off duty, working those days only until six PM. A heavy workload often meant an intern had to forego his time off and remain on duty. For example, one morning during my internship the otolaryngologist had twelve tonsillectomies booked. He was the man who had devised a gadget called the tonsillotome, a combined snare and guillotine that permitted tonsillectomies with a local, rather than general, anaesthetic. We cleared up the twelve operations, he and I taking alternate cases. Then, thinking I had a night off, I climbed on the table to have mine removed. We made some small joke about me being the thirteenth patient. Sent to my room to rest, I was recalled two hours later because of a rush of work. I had to stay on duty all that day and all through my 'night off,' finally returning to my quarters about four PM the next day. Ice cream was all I had been able to eat during the whole time.

Yet it never occurred to us to complain, nor to insist upon our rights under the contract, nor to demand time and a half for overtime. We were still students and learning something every day. One was grateful for the privilege of these experiences, tucking away in the mind bits of knowledge which some day could prove useful.

One experience that interns in most Canadian hospitals miss is riding an ambulance. Few Canadian hospitals have operated ambulances; ambulances are costly items and funds for such a service have not generally been available. My New York internship included four months of riding an ambulance, an experience never to be forgotten.

Memories remain vivid, for instance, of performing a penknife tracheotomy on a child choking with laryngeal diphtheria and of losing the child when the temporary restoration of breathing could not revive a dying heart; of the fury of the packed room of Latin neighbors who saw me 'kill' the child; of their attack and of the help of Tony, my driver, whose flying fists and shouted explanations in fluent Italian allowed me to escape down four flights of stairs to the ambulance with its motor running.

Nor shall I ever forget my daily visits to the narcotics wing of a New York City prison. The howling of the addicts, each wanting to be treated first, was truly heart wrenching. There was a time that I delivered a still-born baby. The distraught father picked up a carving knife yelling, 'Dead bambino, dead doc.' He chased me around front room, back room and hall-way of his flat until I thought of hurling a chair through the front window to attract the attention of the driver and a policeman below. I recall too, the experience of a fellow intern who did a caesarean operation on a dead woman under the wheels of a crosstown streetcar and brought a live baby back to the hospital. Few of today's interns have the opportunity for this breadth of experience.

2

The development of quality care
in hospitals
The basic elements

Patient care of the highest possible quality has been the ultimate objective of all modern hospitals. Advances in medical science, and the dedication and concern of health personnel, produced by a society which puts high priorities on the health and well-being of the individual, are obvious requirements for any substantial long-term improvement in hospital care. In Canada, the organization of hospital services has evolved from a predominantly voluntary basis into a partnership of government and the forces of voluntarism. Each has played a unique and important role in the improvement of hospital standards.

The part played by hospital associations, the development of improved qualifications of hospital personnel and the utilization of insurance principles to make hospital care universally available, are factors so fundamental that they are considered separately in subsequent chapters. Similarly the improvements in the actual physical facilities, outlined in Chapter 6, have had a considerable effect on the quality of care available in hospitals.

THE IMPACT OF MEDICAL SCIENCE

Technology, as applied to the care and treatment of the diseased and disabled has produced a great proliferation of benefits for mankind. Based on the fundamental, invaluable advances made in the nineteenth century and early twentieth century in anatomy, physiology, bacteriology, and pathology, more curative drugs and procedures have been developed in the past twenty years alone than in the whole previous history of healing. In fact, the frontiers of knowledge in every aspect of medicine have expanded dramatically and continue to expand at an apparently accelerating rate. The partial outline in the first chapter of the improved hospital and medical procedures, facilities and services introduced over the past half century have been made possible only by a continuation and extension of ambitious and successful research programs.

Although able to support only a fraction of the worldwide effort in medical research, Canada has nevertheless made important contributions. In 1920, most medical research in Canada was undertaken by a few physicians on medical school teaching staffs working part-time on a shoestring budget. In 1916, when the Honorary Advisory Council for Scientific and Industrial Research (the predecessor of the National Research Council) was formed, 'there were few research laboratories and only a few workers; perhaps some fifty men in the whole of Canada were competent to carry on real research.'[1]

The efforts of even these few men were severely restricted by lack of teamwork and the absence of financial support. Drs Banting, Best and Collip had no Medical Research Council, disease-oriented volunteer agencies or service-club philanthropy to sponsor their efforts. University budgets were tight and the Rockefeller Foundation was only beginning to extend its generous support to Canadian medical schools. The medical researcher usually was faced with personal financial sacrifices.

The discovery of insulin by Banting and Best in 1921 had an immediate and far-reaching effect on medical research in Canada; it stimulated the flow of financial support. The Banting Research Fund, the Commonwealth Fund, the Rockefeller Foundation and others contributed enormously to worthwhile research projects across the country in the 1920s and 1930s. The University of Toronto School of Hygiene, the Banting Institute, the Montreal Neurological Institute and others were established as excellent research centres by 1935.

Not until 1938 did the federal government set up a program explicitly supporting extramural medical research. At that time an Associate Medical Research Committee of the National Research Council was established under the chairmanship of Sir Frederick Banting. The initial budget of $53,000 grew to more than $150,000 in 1946 when the Associate Committee changed its name to the Medical Division of the NRC. Fifteen years later the Medical Research Council was created as a separate entity, independent of the National Research Council.

1 *Report of the Royal Commission on National Development in the Arts, Letters and Sciences* (Ottawa, the King's Printer, 1951), p. 174

Besides the NRC and MRC several other federal departments and agencies have supported medical research. The Defence Research Board, formally established in 1948, has traditionally sponsored research of particular significance to the armed services. The Department of National Health and Welfare, although originally specializing in problems of public health, has greatly expanded its assistance to all types of research programs. The Department of Veterans Affairs has gradually increased its sponsorship of research within its own hospitals, thereby attracting and assisting many members of medical school faculties to do research in problems of chronic illness and care.

Canadian medical research has always relied to some extent on the philanthropy of private individuals and agencies. In addition to the foundations previously mentioned and others, various voluntary societies increased their efforts to raise funds for this purpose, especially after the second world war. The provincial Heart Foundations, the National Cancer Institute, the Canadian Arthritis and Rheumatism Society, the Muscular Dystrophy Association and the Canadian Cystic Fibrosis Foundation are a few outstanding examples.

Provincial governments have jurisdiction over education. In helping to finance medical schools the provinces have sometimes earmarked considerable funds in support of medical research. In addition, some of the indirect costs of research in teaching hospitals have been subsidized in per diem grants. Some provinces have contributed heavily to research-funding agencies or directly sponsored their own research. Occasionally semi-voluntary agencies have been set up by provincial staute and although they may receive much money from the province they usually have substantial alternative sources of revenue. The Addiction Research Foundation, the Cancer Treatment and Research Foundation and the Mental Health Foundation are examples in Ontario. In recent years Ontario and Quebec have centralized and separately budgeted health research grants to some extent.

Despite a remarkable growth in total expenditures, financial support for medical research was deemed alarmingly inadequate by the Association of Canadian Medical Colleges in the late 1950s. As a result of this concern, and the report of the Farquharson committee,[2] the Medical Research Council was split off from the NRC in 1961 with a greatly expanded budget. By 1969–70 the MRC was expending more than thirty million annually on project support, fellowships, associateships, scholarships and travel grants.

2 *Report of the Special Committee Appointed to Review Extramural Support of Medical Research by the Government of Canada*, to the Committee of the Privy Council on Scientific and Industrial Research

In 1965 a further impetus came with the establishment of the federal government's Health Resources Fund to improve teaching and research facilities in medical schools and teaching hospitals.

Another important granting agency since the late fifties has been the National Institutes of Health of the United States Public Health Service.

As a result of these ever-increasing sources of financial support, many thousands of skilled scientists have been able to spend time and effort in medical research. No complete list of Canadian contributions to medical research is available but near the top would be the works of Banting, Best, Collip, Barr and Penfield. There are dozens more who were or are recognized internationally as leaders in their field. For their efforts and achievements Canadians can be justifiably proud.

As a result of medical research the practice of medicine has become much more scientifically sophisticated. Tests and procedures have become more numerous and complex and, as a result, more time-consuming and expensive. Advanced equipment, other facilities and services have become centralized in hospitals, the only institutions that can afford them and ensure their efficient utilization.

In addition medical research has contributed to the improvement of quality care in hospitals by the actual presence of research programs and scientists within or in close proximity to the institution. Most research is undertaken in medical schools, or in some cases in pharmaceutical or government laboratories. A significant portion, however, is concentrated in teaching hospitals. The most obvious reason is the abundance and variety of patients and their meticulously kept records which are essential to clinical investigation.

In no way disparaging the importance of basic research in the pre-clinical sciences, Jacques Genest has observed that:

There is no doubt in the mind of anyone concerned with modern diagnosis and treatment of patients that the quality of medical care in any country is directly proportional to the volume of first-class clinical research conducted in its hospitals and to the extent of the facilities placed at the disposal of its clinical investigators. It is certainly no mere coincidence that the best consultation centres in the world for the diagnosis and treatment of diseases are also those possessing the greatest number of qualified clinical investigators and the more extensive research facilities.[3]

The scientific method, so rigorously upheld and practised in reputable

3 Jacques Genest, 'Clinical Research in Canada,' *Canadian Medical Association Journal*, 14 April 1962, vol. 86, p. 680

research programs, is tremendously contagious. Research creates an atmosphere wherein knowledge is fervently sought and revered. Clinical education for medical students and patient care benefit accordingly. The training received by the majority of physicians at these research centres is ultimately applied to the treatment and care of people in other hospitals and regions.

There has long been a great variation in the scope of research undertaken in teaching hospitals. Some have research institutes with full-time professional and administrative directors and elaborate facilities – for example, the Hospital for Sick Children in Toronto. Others have clinical investigation units with informal professional control and administration. Most teaching hospitals co-operate with medical schools in joint research projects. Small research units in the area of specific interest to the sponsoring voluntary agency are present in many teaching hospitals and are usually supervised by full-time research associates on a local medical faculty staff.

Each hospital has had its own admistrative procedures for facilitating and supervising its research programs. As a rule the hospital administrator has been involved in the research organization only to the extent that material contributions are made by the hospital to research funds and facilities.

Finally, the quality of clinical teaching has tended to vary directly with the amount and quality of research undertaken in a teaching hospital and in the medical school with which the hospital is affiliated. The best teachers, most of whom have varying degrees of interest in research, have been attracted to the institutions with superior research facilities.

The proliferation of hospital personnel and evolution of responsibilities within the hospital (as well as the increasing costs of hospitalization) largely reflect advances in medical science. These and other more complex repercussions of medical technology are discussed in later chapters.

Technology, of course, has never been more than a tool for men to use. Throughout the period 1920 to 1970 it has been used mostly to reinforce the roles that hospitals had already assumed. As the role of the hospital expanded over the years, new technology was devised and utilized to facilitate this expansion.

Only in recent years, with the pressures of rising costs and the need for a more efficient and comprehensive health delivery system, have hospitals incorporated medical technology of a more automated, and therefore more efficient, nature. Monitors, closed-circuit television, computers, multi-test laboratory machines, mobile robots and the like, are increasingly being used for diagnosis and therapy. These innovations often speed up service and can save lives, too, for the human equation is often not so consistently reliable as the mechanical counterpart. More automation of a type which will lower costs appreciably and improve the quality of treatment is imperative.

To be sure, automation, almost by definition, raises various problems of retraining for paramedical and ancillary staff. But the real dangers lie in introducing it indiscriminately in patient-contact areas. Before proceeding further in this respect we must be careful to introduce measures to ensure that patient care does not become too depersonalized or even partially sacrificed to economic gain.

SPECIALIZATION IN MEDICINE
THE ROYAL COLLEGE OF PHYSICIANS AND SURGEONS
OF CANADA

An inevitable consequence of the rapid growth of medical knowledge and technology has been increasing specialization in all areas of health care, especially in the practice of medicine.

The question of what constituted a specialist was still a perplexing problem in the twenties for the simple reason that no generally acceptable Canadian standard existed. If a man had returned from London or Edinburgh with an FRCS, he was quickly recognized. If he had an MRCP or, better, the far-from-common FRCP, he was accepted as a qualified internist. The fellowship of the American College of Surgeons (FACS), a degree of more recent development, was not as readily recognized (by the holders of the FRCS, in particular) because it was based more on practical experience and ability than upon a detailed knowledge of the basic medical sciences. The FACS, however, were competent surgeons and many built substantial practices. Holders of postgraduate degrees in obstetrics were most frequently connected with the teaching hospitals. In the more limited clinical specialties, such as orthopaedics, ophthalmology or otolaryngology, it was largely a matter of having served an extended internship or residency on such special service, sometimes in Canada, more often in Great Britain, the U.S., or in France, often with an intensive course in certain special areas in Vienna. Most surgeons were general surgeons, even though especially qualified or proficient in a special area. Internists, too, were general internists to a large extent. In the larger hospitals they may have been neurologists, gastroenterologists, cardiologists, or pulmonary specialists, but these terms had not become a part of public language. Actually internists had difficulty practising as internists anywhere outside of the larger urban centres.

The profession recognized them but, to the average family, they were just doctors who didn't operate or deliver babies. It was frequently difficult for such a specialist to get more than a general practitioner's fee on direct office visits or even on consultations. Dermatologists were consulted directly, but allergists, haematologists, endocrinologists and others practising subspecialties did so usually as an adjunct to their normal practice in a broader specialty.

Paediatricians usually had served an internship in a children's hospital and then stayed on for further experience. Others with more limited internship often developed large practices in smaller centres as an offshoot of general practice. Dr Alan Brown, the dynamic and greatly respected ruler of the Hospital for Sick Children in Toronto, lived to see a remarkable number of the top positions in paediatrics in various Canadian and American centres filled by his former residents. I once asked him the secret of his large private practice. He replied facetiously, 'I was the first doctor in the province to install in my office suite a child-sized toilet; the children wanted to come back just to use it again.'

A large percentage of the specialists of the day, and those frequently called in by the family physicians on consultation, were former general practitioners themselves who had become specialists by virtue of hard work, learning by experience and developing a great fund of practical knowledge. Many were excellent, used good judgment, got good results and knew when to call in someone more experienced; others, unfortunately, could not be so characterized.

To the Canadian public (in contrast to the attitude in Great Britain), the qualification of the specialist meant little. When a specialist was needed, the choice was left to the family doctor or the recommendation of a neighbour was accepted. Dr Herbert A. Bruce, an outstanding surgeon, founder and surgeon-in-chief of the Wellesley Hospital in Toronto, was already a legendary character in my boyhood. Although I do not remember actually seeing it, I have retained a vivid mental picture of the young surgeon on his way to a day's work – yellow gloved, holding a tight rein on his spirited team of horses, heading south from Rosedale, across the bridge and down well-gravelled Jarvis St past the homes of Sir William Mulock and the other elite of the day. Was it not routine for Dr Bruce to remove an appendix with total elapsed time of seven minutes from the first incision to the final stitch? Or was it five? Or four? What careers have been made or broken over the bridge table and the garden fence.

Fee-splitting, or dichotomy, had been prevalent before the first world war and had still not entirely died out in the 1920s. The practice had arisen because of the feeling on the part of many general practitioners that there was too big a gap between the fee of the surgeon and that of the family doctor who had carried the burden of diagnosing the case, getting consent for surgery, making the arrangements, often assisting and then carrying through the post-operative period. It is not the function of this book to debate the issue which is now a matter of the past. However, it can be said that fee-splitting did develop large practices for a number of surgeons, which were not always the sole result of their particular surgical abilities.

Before specialty qualifications were defined with some precision, the larger public hospitals, and some smaller ones too, were exercising commendable judgment in controlling the actions of individual staff members. Legal action was rare in the twenties partly because the right of the board to take disciplinary action was very clear in those cases which reached the court. Also, no board acted precipitously; justification for the action was usually quite obvious by the time action was taken.

Our larger cities then had more private hospitals than now. These were largely used for medical cases, obstetrics and a certain amount of less-than-exacting surgery. Their equipment was more limited than that of the public hospitals and their requirements respecting the qualification of their nurses, their medical records, and so on, left much to be desired. While some excellent doctors with public hospital appointments used these hospitals (their patient charges were usually lower or it may have been a matter of convenience), they were also used by doctors with limited or no connections with the public hospitals. Sometimes the very existence of private hospitals in a situation that lacked governmental control made it difficult for the public hospital to protect the public.

For instance, while on the teaching staff of the Toronto Western Hospital I was instructed, as secretary of the medical staff, to inform a certain doctor with an itchy scalpel finger that he could no longer perform major surgery in the hospital. Infuriated, he declared that he would take his work to a private hospital where they had 'no such silly regulations.' And he did.

What was badly needed in Canada was a hallmark of recognition for qualified specialists, a standard that would be Canadian and not necessarily involve recognition by bodies in other countries. At the 1920 meeting of the Canadian Medical Association, Dr Sam Moore of Regina proposed that steps be taken to set up a Canadian Royal College of Surgeons and Physicians.[4] Opinion was divided concerning the timeliness of the proposal

4 Sclater Lewis, *The Royal College of Physicians and Surgeons of Canada 1920 to 1960* (McGill University Press, 1962), p. 5, and T.C. Routley, 'The founding of the Royal College of Physicians and Surgeons of Canada,' *Report of Annual Meeting and Proceedings*, 1954

or what body would sponsor it. However by 1926 a proposal by a CMA committee under Dr Prowse of Winnipeg was approved and a working party under Dr David Low of Regina and later under Dr F.N.G. Starr with Dr T.C. Routley as secretary worked out the innumerable details. The next step was to get parliamentary sanction which in turn required provincial approval. It was a painstaking procedure strewn with difficulties. However, authority was finally obtained and the initial meeting of the Royal College of Physicians and Surgeons of Canada was held on November 20, 1929. At this meeting Dr Jonathan C. Meakins, professor of medicine at McGill University, was elected president, with Dr T.C. Routley as secretary pro tem.

The charter members were the 'professors in medicine, surgery, gynaecology or obstetrics in a Canadian university.' The charter provided that others who were selected as fellows within two years would also be considered charter members. Difficult situations arose because not all medical schools used the same titles for heads of specialty divisions. What about an assistant professorship? And who should be selected among the leading doctors of cities and regions without medical schools? It was an interesting time to be in the CMA office – without responsibility for these particular headaches.

Since those early days the college has come a long way. Today, specialty examinations are held for two types of candidates: (a) for fellowship, in seventeen specialties in medicine and ten in surgery; (b) for certification (since 1946), in eleven specialties in medicine and six in surgery. Approval has been given to specialist qualification in respiratory disease and in rheumatology but examinations have not been conducted as yet.[5] As of May 1971, there were 5,493 fellows; in addition there were 8,982 specialists in Canada certified by the Royal College; this makes a total of 14,475 Canadian physicians and surgeons who hold Royal College specialty certification. This figure is only slightly less than one-half of the total physician population of the country.

In recent years the Royal College formulated plans to conduct but one examination – for certification.[6] Successful candidates may then, or later, be elected to fellowship in the college.

The clarification of who is and who is not a specialist did a great deal to simplify the problem of granting hospital privileges for specialized work. During the transition some heartaches resulted when hospitals adopted the requirement of certification and limited the work of some excellent sur-

5 The first examinations were conducted in 1972.
6 This new system was established, as planned, in 1972.

geons whose ability came from long experience, not certification. However, evaluation of a movement must be on its long-range implications, not solely on its effect on individuals during the transition period. Already certification has more than justified its implementation.

The approval of hospitals for residency in the various approved specialties has been another beneficial effect of the work of the Royal College. Beginning in 1956 standards for each specialty program were established. Instead of haphazard apprenticeships to leading specialists, the residencies have become well organized, more educational than in the past, and carefully checked by an approval committee.

In addition to an approved internship, candidates for College certification must have completed four more years of graduate training. This is normally spent in hospitals, one year in the general subject (medicine or surgery) as a resident, two years in the specialty concerned, and a fourth year on an optional subject. This procedure varies somewhat with the specialty; for instance, a candidate must have spent in ophthalmology one year of internship, one in medicine or surgery and three years in ophthalmology. Some hospital departments receive varying levels of approval depending upon their ability to train the resident – periods of approval that vary from six months to full training.

However, the major change in recent years is that most of these postgraduate training courses are now under the direction of university faculties of medicine, a considerable change and improvement from the days when most of the medical faculties took little or no responsibility for graduate training.

THE STANDARDIZATION-ACCREDITATION PROGRAM

Without question one of the greatest single influences in bringing about a high level of medical care in our general hospitals was the standardization program initiated by the American College of Surgeons. As the twenties dawned it was apparent to the members of both the u.s. and Canadian organizations that the time had come when something had to be done to improve the facilities of many hospitals. Further, it was obvious that hospitals required better staff organization and more clinical controls. The obvious approach was to set up standards by which a hospital's degree of efficiency could be measured.

When this movement was launched in 1918 and 1919, Dr Franklin H. Martin was the secretary-general of the American College. Dr Martin was a dynamic and imaginative individual who was ably supported by a board which included Doctors George Crile of Cleveland, Lahey of Boston, Ochsner of New Orleans and other leading surgeons. The standardization requirements[7] included many items which were in the interests of both the patients and better medical service.

Written pre-operative diagnoses were required to reduce hasty surgery without a careful diagnostic study. The details of each operation were to be carefully recorded. Anaesthetists were to be better qualified. The hospital was required to have a satisfactory laboratory department run by a competent pathologist and an adequate radiological department supervised by an acceptable radiologist. The clinical records of all patients were to be completed; deliquent doctors were to have their hospital privileges suspended until the records were brought up to date. Staff meetings were to be held monthly with a review of all hospital deaths. Later, tumor, tissue and other committees were required. Data was checked with respect to autopsy findings and the percentage of autopsies in relation to the number of deaths. The qualifications of technicians, the appointment of a trained dietitian to supervise the food service and other indications of superior care and efficiency were closely scrutinized.

Hospitals were either 'approved,' 'provisionally approved' or 'not approved.' The movement got off to a shaky start but was soon recognized as one of the greatest milestones in hospital development.

The standardization program was a bold and imaginative step but it required a genius with unbounded energy to implement it. The college found its genius in Dr Malcolm T. MacEachern, a Canadian who had been born at Woodville, Ontario, near Lindsay, who had trained at McGill and who, in 1918, was superintendent of the Vancouver General Hospital.

When he joined the ACS standardization committee, Dr MacEachern moved to Chicago but his heart remained in Canada. Provincial conventions and Canadian problems had high priority on his busy schedule. With Matthew Foley, editor of *Hospital Management* and father of the annual 'Hospital Day,' Dr MacEachern created the American College of Hospital Administrators, an organization which has lived up to the enthusiastic vision of its founders. It was his inspiration that created the college's code of ethics and he was instrumental in getting the American Hospital Association to adopt the same code.

More than anything else, Dr MacEachern saw that to be successful the standardization procedures for hospitals had to be explained to, and understood by, the public. Each year at the annual meeting of the American Col-

7 See Appendix A.

lege of Surgeons, Dr MacEachern would arrange a public meeting at which the procedures would be explained, in layman's language, to the public.

I recall one such meeting in St Louis where more than 3,000 persons were turned away from the packed convention hall. Dr MacEachern had a showman's touch in organizing these public meetings. Bob Jolly, a former evangelist and gospel singer who was a hospital administrator from Houston, would 'warm up' the audience with humorous anecdotes and stories about doctors and medicine. Then a 'name' personality – perhaps Dr Charles Mayo or Dr George Crile – would explain new developments in medicine. A hospital trustee or administrator would follow with an explanation of the standardization program. Dr MacEachern's plan worked: the ACS plan to impose standards on North American hospitals got tremendous press and radio coverage, and the public was made aware of its need.

During the time he was organizing the standardization program, Dr MacEachern was also writing *Hospital Organization and Management*,[8] a book which was to become the bible for North American Hospital administrators. MacEachern was an early riser – he was usually out of bed by five AM to personally assess standardization reports on various hospitals. During the two years his book was in the works, he rose at four AM to get an extra hour for writing. It was a gruelling routine for him and imposed a strain on lesser mortals (like me) who travelled with him and had to listen to the shuffling of papers and the sharpening of pencils at an hour when I wanted desperately to be asleep.

It is possible that almost everyone who bears a name with the prefix Mac- is known to his friends, naturally, as 'Mac.' But during the early years of the standardization program, there was no one in the North American hospital field who could have doubted who you spoke of when you mentioned the name, Dr Mac. The Sisters of the religious hospitals adored him. With no disrespect to the Sisters, he was their pin-up man; many a Sister told me she treasured a small picture of Dr MacEachern among her few personal possessions. Father Alphonse Schwitalla, the brilliant and witty president of the Catholic Hospital Association of the United States and Canada,

8 In the foreword of this book I had the privilege of writing the following words about its author, a judgment I have never had cause to re-assess: 'There is general agreement that no one individual has ever amassed such a wealth of experience with hospital problems, has ever has such first hand knowledge of so many hospitals and acquaintance with their personnel, has ever received so many calls for advice, has ever contributed in so many ways towards higher standards of hospital efficiency, nor has so consistently sacrificed himself to the ceaseless demands of his beloved and appreciative hospital and medical colleagues.'

once 'complained' to a hospital meeting: 'Although I am supposed to be head of the Catholic hospitals of this continent, the Sisters call me simply, "Father Schwitalla." Dr MacEachern, however, is known as "Pope MacEachern".'

In 1939 the American Hospital Association established its highest award, the annual Award of Merit, and MacEachern was its first recipient. (Five years earlier, the AHA had awarded a special merit citation to Matthew Foley.) Appropriately enough, the meeting at which Dr MacEachern's award was presented was held in Canada. Dr MacEachern was a humble man but he cherished with justifiable pride a chain of golden keys, each one of which represented an honor or a membership in some professional association. He always wore the chain – hung under his lapel.

Dr MacEachern's work on the standardization procedures made him the best known, most widely travelled and best informed individual in the North American hospital field. In time, his reputation and fame was known around the world.

But in the early years of the standardization and accreditation program many problems were encountered, some not anticipated. It was not difficult to interest the hospital trustees who, naturally, wanted their pride and joy on any approved list. The biggest difficulty arose with individual doctors.

The doctors were busy and tired. The insistence on writing up records was ridiculous; they had their office records – and, to be fair, some actually had. An 'exploratory' laparotomy did not put one's diagnostic ability to a test as did a written pre-operative diagnosis that others could later check. Laboratory tests were unreliable; (here, the objecting doctors often had a point, for the lab technicians seldom had enough supervised training or experience and their reagents often were not accurately made). The doctors said they were too busy for staff meetings and few wanted to curry disfavor by sitting on committees critical of others. On the Prairies, in particular, the doctors took pride in all being on the same level. All were licensed to practise surgery and who among them would deny another the privilege? Many a doctor, to my personal knowledge, protested any kind of supervisory committee and refused to serve.

Some medical staffs were downright hostile to the standardization program and to anyone introducing it, despite the fact that the Canadian Medical Association at its 1921 meeting had given 'unqualified approval of the plan of standardization for the hospitals of the Dominion.' On one occasion Dr MacEachern and I were going to a meeting of the medical staff of an active, city-owned hospital in the west. He had to face a hostile medical staff that planned to dissociate itself from 'standardization.' I had to face the same staff, a group of men smarting from press criticisms arising from published excerpts of a study I had made which revealed many of their serious inadequacies.

In those days, travel was largely by train and Dr MacEachern and I travelled many thousands of miles together, en route to conventions, conferences or medical staff meetings.

On this occasion, when we alighted from the train, we were met by a friendly member of the medical staff of the hospital we were to visit. He advised us to climb back aboard the train and continue west since he knew that a few of his confreres had hinted that for Dr MacEachern a suitable welcome would consist of tar and feathers.

We elected to stay.

It was a cold night but the icicles inside the meeting hall were longer than those without. I spoke first and hoped I could clarify the misunderstanding. The board of this municipal hospital had asked for a frank appraisal of its physical facilities and administrative setup. Everyone knew the buildings were obsolete and the management needing shaking up. But the board did not realize how truly disintegrated the situation had become until I submitted my report. While preparing the report, the executive committee of the medical staff asked me if I would include a chapter appraising the staffing arrangements 'and don't pull any punches'. I was as frank as they requested.

After my report had been submitted to the board, the local press asked the board for a copy which was being kept confidential. Finally, someone on the board or someone at city hall leaked the final chapter only, the one relating to the medical staff. Most of the doctors, not knowing of their executive's request, assumed this was the whole of an unasked-for report – and reacted accordingly. That night, when the doctors saw the whole report, their attitude changed at once. They even applauded when they heard excerpts from the unpublished chapters.

I weathered my personal storm but Dr MacEachern had a rougher time. He was asking them, in essence, to increase greatly their joint and individual responsibility for the quality of service given to the patients. He was asking busy men to give more of their time to non-remunerative hospital work and to risk friendships by sitting in judgment on each other. This he did in a diplomatic and logical way, always maintaining as the one goal the best interests of the patient. Soon he had members of the audience answering the criticisms and strongly supporting the standardization requirements. Before the meeting closed, the medical staff endorsed standardization by an almost unanimous vote. Moreover, before they left, every last man in the hall lined up to shake Dr MacEachern's hand.

A major reason for the rapid acceptance of hospital standardization despite opposition such as this was the assistance given by the Reverend Father Moulinier on behalf of the Catholic Hospital Association of the United States and Canada. Many of the towns and smaller cities of Canada had two hospitals, one a Catholic hospital operated by Sisters and the other non-denominational and operated either by a voluntary board of trustees or by the municipality. Many medical staffs were either sceptical or opposed to the concept of standardization. In the case of the Sisters' hospitals, the orders had a considerable influence on the individual hospital's policies. Thanks to Father Moulinier's influence, the Sisters' hospital in quite a number of communities became the first to be standardized. When this was announced in the press, citizens began to ask why the other hospital, often tax-supported, did not have the same efficiency rating, although both hospitals often shared the same medical staff. These pressures began to bring results.

The American College of Surgeons carried on the full program of accreditation from 1919 to 1951, a tremendous undertaking and a formidable expense. The cost and the absorption of staff time became so burdensome by the late forties that the college began to question the wisdom of bearing the whole expense itself. With the retirement of Dr MacEachern, the shift to more shoulders became necessary. Much discussion among the national medical and hospital bodies ensued; at one time, it appeared that the American Medical Association might take over. American hospitals which did not want accreditation to be subject to some current pressures by the organized profession opposed the move. It was finally agreed that several medical and hospital bodies (ACS, AMA, AHA, and ACP) would participate in a Joint Commission on the Accreditation of Hospitals (JCAH). In 1953 the JCAH invited the CMA to send a representative and to facilitate the continued existence of the standardization-accreditation program in Canada; Canadian doctors accepted.

The joint commission began to take over accreditation in December 1951 under the direction of Dr Edwin L. Crosby, later executive director (and subsequently executive president) of the American Hospital Association and president in the late 1960s of the International Hospital Federation. Three years later, when Dr Crosby left for the AHA, Dr Kenneth B. Babcock took over and directed the work of the joint commission until 1965 when he was succeeded by Dr John D. Porterfield.

Coincident with the development of the JCAH in the U.S. was the rise of a Canadian movement for a separate accreditation program in Canada. Beginning at the CMA annual meeting in 1950 in Halifax, a Committee on the Accreditation of Hospitals was established, under the chairmanship of Dr Kirk Lyon of Leamington, Ontario. This shortly expanded into the Canadian Commission on Hospital Accreditation with representation from the CMA, CHA, RCPS and l'Association des Médécins de Langue Française du Canada. Although the ultimate objective of this commission was to create and operate a separate Canadian hospital accreditation program, financial, personnel and related problems delayed the realization of his objective throughout most of the fifties. By a special 1955 arrangement the majority of JCAH Canadian surveys were, in fact, done by Dr Karl Hollis, Dr J.J. Laurier and others who were directly responsible to the Canadian Commission on Hospital Accreditation. By mid-1958, due largely to the efforts and perseverance of men such as Dr Kirk Lyon, Dr A.D. Kelly of the Canadian Medical Association, Dr L.O. Bradley, Rev Hector Bertrand and others, obstacles had been overcome and an agreement was negotiated with the JCAH whereby the Canadian body, subsequently known as the Canadian Council on Hospital Accreditation, assumed complete responsibility and control of the accreditation program in Canada on January 1, 1959.

If the spirits of those who have departed can rise up and dance on their graves, there must have been gay shenanigans in one or more cemeteries in the Regina area on that New Year's Day of 1959. The plan adopted was precisely what the Regina nucleus of doctors wanted back in 1929 when they supported the CMA's decision to set up a Department of Hospital Service to help the hospitals in their many problems. Drs David Low, Sam Moore and Dave Johnson wanted a completely separate Canadian approval body, one that would be less strict about written records and one that would generally set standards to suit Canadian conditions. I had just left a clinical and teaching career to take over this work and I was as admantly opposed to the all-Canadian concept as they were in favor. 'Sometime in the future but the time is not yet ripe.' Thirty-one years later what they wanted did take place – the time was ripe. At least a separate body was set up. The requirements, however, were not eased; if anything, they were and are more exacting.

Dr Karl E. Hollis, former Officer Commanding the hospital ship *Lady Nelson* and administrator of Sunnybrook (DVA) Hospital, and Dr J.J. Laurier were appointed surveyors in 1954, Dr Hollis retiring in 1957 because of ill health. In 1957, Dr William I. Taylor was appointed director of the Canadian program and he was succeeded in 1969 by Dr Leonard O. Bradley.

The members of the CCHA at the time of the inauguration of the Canadian program in 1959 were: CHA *representatives*: Dr Austin M. Clarke, Moncton, NB; Dr J.E.G. Lasalle, Montreal; Dr J.B. Neilson, Toronto; Rev A.L. Danis, Ottawa; J.E. Robinson, Winnipeg. CMA *representatives*: Dr E. Kirk Lyon, Leamington, Ont.; Dr D.A. Thompson, Bathurst, NB; Dr N.N. Levinne, Toronto; Dr B.H. McNeel, Toronto. RCPS(C) *representatives*: Dr A.L. Chute (CCHA chairman), Toronto; Dr W.K. Welch, Toronto. *L'Association des Médécins de Langue Française du Canada representative*: Dr E. Thibault, Verdun, Que.

By 1970 a total of 525 hospitals in Canada had entered the accreditation program. This represented 131,585 beds out of a total in all hospitals of 212,354 beds, or 61.5 percent. The great majority of the medium-sized and larger active treatment hospitals are approved, the lag being in the smaller hospitals,[9] in extended care facilities, and in mental and psychiatric institutions of which only seven of 116 were in the program. Generally only a very small proportion of hospitals surveyed or resurveyed have not been accredited.

The standards in recent years have been less rigid although no less exacting. The standards are interpreted in relation to the resources available in the community and the arrangements made for provision of services not available in the region.

THE VOLUNTARY AGENCIES

To serve one's fellow man has long been the prime motivation of millions of people performing dedicated service to aid the diseases and disabled. Often reinforced by religious tenets and a philosophic optimism, the spirit of voluntarism has pervaded the delivery of health care around the world.

In Canada the earliest hospitals were run under the auspices of the Catholic Sisters. Originally conceived to provide for the spiritual and religious needs of the sick, Catholic hospitals were traditionally founded under the authority of the bishop of the diocese and run as charitable institutions.

One of my very pleasant memories of the late thirties centres on the tercentenary celebration of the Hôtel Dieu of Quebec, the oldest hospital north of Mexico. The eleven-day celebration was remarkable. The oldest part of the present hospital had been erected in 1696, replacing earlier destroyed buildings, and those of us who visited the cloister could see old

---

9 Active treatment hospitals with fewer than twenty-five beds and fewer than three member on the medical staff, as well as all extended care hospitals, became eligible for accreditation in 1970.

bullet marks on the walls and the candle-lit cells still in use. Framed registries of the early nuns indicated that some of those Sisters had spent fifty, sixty, seventy and in one instance seventy-six years in this cloister. Near the garden exit was the tiny room where the Sisters worshipped during the siege of Quebec in 1759. At the 1939 celebration the cloistered Augustine and Ursuline Sisters had the unique experience of leaving the hospital confines and walking nearly two hundred-strong to the Pontifical Mass in the Basilica.

Illustrious guests from many parts of the world attended and were received by His Eminence Cardinal Villeneuve. Among those taking part was Father Alphonse Schwitalla, president of the Catholic Hospital Association of the United States and Canada, who presented four large volumes of testimonials from some six hundred hospitals in the two countries. The whole celebration was a tribute to the organizing ability of the sisters, to Dr Charles Vezina, the surgeon-in-chief, and to the hospital celebrations committee. The Quebec government helped to sponsor the event with a donation of $100,000.

Since the founding of this original hospital in 1639, Catholic hospitals have proliferated across Canada and the United States. By 1920 there were more than one hundred in Canada alone. For many years the Sisters' orders have operated about one-third of the voluntary hospitals in Canada. These have included institutions of all types and sizes from the enormous mental institutions – St Michel Archange in Quebec and St Jean de Dieu in Montreal – to small community hospitals in almost all other areas of the country. Many Sisters' orders provided the only hospital care available in some regions. Of the Sisters' selfless devotion to their work one writer has said:

In founding the new hospitals in the western part of the country special credit must be given to the religious communities of eastern Canada who willingly and generously supplied the necessary religious to undertake the work. In many cases, especially during the depression years, in addition to supplying the staff, it was necessary for them to subsidize the newly founded hospitals from their common funds in order to make sure that the people of these areas would have the service which the hospitals could provide.[10]

In 1930 a survey conducted by the Catholic Hospital Association listed 134 Catholic hospitals in Canada run by a total of twenty-nine different orders

10 Rev M.C. Doyle, *The Story of the Catholic Hospitals of Canada*, p. 42

of nuns. The major orders were the Grey Nuns, the Sisters of Providence, the Sisters of St Joseph and the Sisters of Misericorde.

Impressive though their efforts were, the Catholic orders could only partially fulfill the hospital needs of the country. To fill the gap hospitals were established by local non-profit hospital associations. In some cases the board of trustees that ran the hospital were elected by a community. In others anyone who contributed a stipulated donation to the hospital and paid an annual fee became a trustee. More typically, however, the board usually re-elected a portion of its membership at stated intervals, the other members being elected from community or government agencies. This is still the procedure most followed by non-sectarian general hospitals.

The local municipal government often gained the right to appoint trustees if it contributed toward capital costs or toward the care of indigents in the hospital.

Regardless of how they are appointed or elected, trustees have traditionally given long, hard hours of labor for their hospital without remuneration. In addition, numerous trustees have been active in hospital associations and in many instances have made remarkable contributions to the hospital system as a whole.

By the early years of this century other organized religious and charitable groups had established hospitals and outposts in urban centres, in rural towns and in destitute regions where health facilities were non-existent. The Methodist (later United) and Anglican Churches, the IODE, the Salvation Army and others were active in this way. Although the hospitals operated by these groups were not numerous they did fill many gaps in the health and hospital care available. Of particular interest are the International Grenfell Association and the Canadian Red Cross Society.

The Grenfell Hospitals of Newfoundland
The story of hospital development in Newfoundland differs considerably from that in other parts of the country. None of the colonial powers – principally Britain and France – which at various times held the island was interested in developing it. Newfoundland, with its rugged coastline, was convenient as a way-stop for the fishing fleets or naval ships; beyond that it held little interest for the larger powers. As a result the island was late in starting any program of hospital building and even today lags behind other provinces. A century ago, when the island's population was approximately one hundred and fifty thousand, Newfoundland had only one small general hospital in St John's, one so-called fever hospital, and an asylum for the insane. There were no hospitals outside the capital and medical conditions in the isolated outports were often desperate.

In 1892, Dr (later Sir) Wilfred Grenfell came to Newfoundland and a new era began. He set up hospitals at Battle Harbour in Labrador in 1893 and at Indian Harbour the following year. The main hospital at St Anthony at the northern tip of Newfoundland's 'finger' was built in 1904 and has continued as a modern, fully accredited hospital doing an amazing range of major work as I can personally testify. Additional hospitals were opened at North West River and Cartwright on the Labrador coast, as were nursing stations at various other coastal points. A hospital ship was outfitted and visited isolated ports. Ancillary services were developed – orphanages, boarding schools, libraries, clothing distribution centres and the teaching of handicrafts.

In 1920 I had the great privilege of meeting Dr Grenfell while he was on a fund-raising campaign in the northeast United States. This legendary rugged individual exuded a missionary zeal and contagious enthusiasm and it was immediately obvious why his hospitals had succeeded so well. Grenfell and his successors have continued to provide a high calibre of health care down through the years in the remote northern settlements. In 1970 the International Grenfell Association maintained five hospitals and twelve nursing outposts in northern Newfoundland and along the Labrador coast.

The Canadian Red Cross Society
Hospital services across the country have been much indebted to the Canadian Red Cross Society over the fifty-year period we are discussing. Apart from its great contribution to the armed forces during both wars, the Red Cross has made two magnificent contributions to hospital care in Canada – the outpost hospital-nursing station program and the Red Cross blood transfusion service.

Responding to the needs of thousands of ex-servicemen and new immigrants settling in pioneer regions of the country far from medical personnel and service, the Canadian Red Cross Society initiated its outpost hospital service in 1920. In co-operation with the Soldier Settlement Board, the provincial Red Cross divisions of Alberta, Saskatchewan, Manitoba and, somewhat later, Ontario, assessed the medical requirements of their sparsely populated regions. Subsequently, beginning in Altario, Alberta, a number of small outpost hospitals and nursing stations were set up. The nurses attached to the smaller units provided a variety of public health services as well as caring for emergencies.

Spreading rapidly in the Prairies and, after 1922, throughout Ontario, the movement had developed into thirty-two units by 1925. While in some provinces certain hospitals were transferred to local control, the movement expanded in others, and by 1940 the Red Cross was operating fifty outposts. This remarkable and sustained growth was due in large measure to the dedicated leadership of the Red Cross provincial divisions and the members of the national Standing Committee (later Advisory Committee) on Outposts. This Committee was formed in 1925 and included Mrs H.P. Plumptre (Ontario), Mrs C.B. Waagen (Alberta), Miss M.E. Wilkinson (Ontario), F.J.L. Harrison (Manitoba), W.F. Kerr (Saskatchewan), Dr Ruggles George (national headquarters) and Dr F.W. Routley, who was chairman of this committee as well as serving as Ontario Red Cross director from 1922 and as national commissioner after 1938. Albert H. Abbott, as general secretary of the Canadian Red Cross Society from 1922 to 1925, and Dr J.L. Biggar, as national commissioner from 1926 to 1937, travelled a great deal across the country promoting and encouraging outpost services.

Perhaps our deepest admiration and gratitude should be directed toward the outpost nurses who served so well under primitive and often frustrating conditions. Physicians, regional or Red Cross, only intermittently visited some of the outposts; in most locations doctors were on hand for only a few weeks each year. Even today, with the traditional outpost image of the small log cabin in the bush largely only a memory, the outpost nurse is called upon to perform a variety of tasks and assume a burden of responsibilities never expected of nurses in heavily populated areas of the country.

By 1929 national Red Cross policy stated that the Society would establish and operate an outpost only at the request of a group, preferably a local Red Cross branch, in the community to be served. The community was expected to carry as much of the costs of building and maintaining the facility as it could and to assume complete control and responsibility as soon as possible. With rare exceptions the Red Cross would not build or administer a hospital of more than twenty beds in the belief that a community so large as to require more than that number of beds should and could support its own facilities. Thus, as communities and regions grew in population and wealth, the Red Cross transferred control of facilities to the communities or community organizations.

For twenty-five years Helen McArthur was National Director of Nursing Services for the Canadian Red Cross Society. A graduate of the University of Alberta, she started her career the hard way by spending three years in the Peace River, handling obstetrics and many of the emergencies herself and learning about the rigors of pioneer life and travel in bitter winter weather. The nursing services of the Canadian Red Cross Society owe much to the leadership over the years of this tall, lissome 'Canadian Nightingale,' as she has been called. In between duties in Canada she played a major part in the rebuilding of the Korean Red Cross and, at one time, was director of the School for Nursing at the University of Alberta. Among her many honors have been the presidency of the Canadian Nurses Association in 1950–54, an honorary LL D from the University of Alberta, the Florence Nightingale Medal (1957), the highest nursing award of the International Red Cross, and the first CNA medal for leadership in the profession. Miss McArthur retired in 1971.

During the second world war the Society expended most of its efforts overseas and in the blood transfusion campaigns. As a result, there was some consolidation and contraction of outpost services. After 1946, however, the Red Cross dramatically expanded outpost facilities until by 1950 there were units operating in eighty-seven Canadian communities. At that time, and until 1958, with the Red Cross paying up to one-third of building costs and operating subsidies, the outposts were the Society's second most expensive service, after the blood transfusion program.

Since that time, with increased financial support from governments to hospitals and improved roads, the number of communities able to operate their hospitals without outside assistance grew and so decreased the need for Red Cross participation ...[11]

By 1957, with the introduction of government-sponsored hospital insurance in all provinces, the Red Cross was able to transfer hospitals to community control. However, in Ontario the provincial government requested the Red Cross to continue to administer the outposts and subsidized the Society in this work. By 1970 there were still twenty-seven outposts in operation in Canada – twelve hospitals in Ontario, four nursing stations in New Brunswick, seven nursing stations in British Columbia, three nursing stations in Quebec and one nursing station in Saskatchewan.

An important side effect of the decision by the Red Cross to continue administration of outpost hospitals in Ontario has been the development and maintenance of an exemplary group of small hospitals. With extensive renovations and rebuilding during the 1960s, efficient and effective administration from division headquarters, and the concern and *esprit de corps* of the society and its members, the outpost hospitals have become, for their size, among the best in the country.

An extension of the traditional role of the Canadian Red Cross Society that brought its services right to the operating room table of every active

11 'Red Cross Outposts in Canada', an unpublished summary by Helen G. McArthur, 1965

treatment hospital in the country, was the Society's undertaking to supply blood, free of charge, to every hospital patient in need.

Blood transfusion became a valued arm of treatment during the first world war with the recognition of different blood groupings. Dr Bruce Robertson of the Hospital for Sick Children, Toronto, made a signal contribution to this subject during the war, as also did Dr Norman M. Guiou of Ottawa, who developed a quick compatibility test using one's spectacles for emergency testing in the trenches. Hospitals used transfusions to good advantage between the wars but there was always the delay of rounding up relatives and friends for blood compatibility tests or of keeping up-to-date lists of professional donors. Almost invariably there was a potentially dangerous time lag. A common hospital requirement was that the family was to furnish two bottles of blood for every bottle of blood used, or pay twenty-five dollars for every bottle used without replacement. It was an expensive procedure, particularly if large amounts were required as in burn cases, severe hemorrhage and some types of surgery. In some provinces the arrangements, including knowledgeable personnel, were quite inadequate.

During the first world war the Red Cross collected more than 2.5 million bottles of blood. There was considerable pressure upon the CRCS towards the end of the war to extend its transfusion service to the civilian hospitals of Canada. Under the chairmanship of Dr John T. Phair, the Society's National Blood and Blood Substitute Committee conducted a survey of civilian hospital requirements. The study, completed in October, 1945, revealed a tremendous need for a nation-wide blood service. The Society developed a plan to supply whole blood, dried plasma (with distilled water for its reconstitution) and sterile administration sets to every hospital in Canada. Central depot laboratories directed from headquarters would be set up across the country; provincial departments of health were asked to provide and maintain these depots. Blood banks were established in all hospitals with major emergency and surgical needs; smaller hospitals would draw from these sources as required. A National Blood Donor Committee was set up under the chairmanship of Harold H. Leather, MBE, and a National Scientific Advisory Committee under Dr John T. Phair. Later a Blood Transfusion Service Policy Committee was established with George Aitken as first chairman. Dr W.S. Stanbury was director of the program for some years.

One stipulation the Society laid down was that the blood it supplied to hospitals should be administered to patients free of charge. While not immediately obvious, this stipulation created a hardship for the hospitals.

For one thing, even if the hospital received the blood (or plasma) free, administering the blood to a patient cost the hospital money and time, linen and so on. A study by the Canadian Hospital Council showed the average cost to the hospitals was about five dollars per transfusion. (Today, of course, such costs are included in the hospital's budget submitted to hospital insurance authorities.) However, it was finally decided not to make this a major issue and the hospitals agreed to absorb the extra costs as best they could.

The results of this service have been striking. From 1947 to 1970 more than 13 million bottles of blood were collected and millions of patients received free transfusions. In 1970 alone the number of units of blood collected was 953,053 and 237,439 patients received transfusions. In the beginning most cross-matching was done at the collecting depots. By 1970 more than ninety percent was done by the participating hospitals, a further yardstick of the extent to which the hospitals have shared with the Red Cross in making this service free to the patients. Rare sub-types, when not at the hospital, are obtained by the Red Cross from other areas by car or even plane and often with the aid of the police.

A life-saving service like this can be used prodigally. In some hospitals the surgeons have prescribed blood almost routinely and certainly very freely. As a result, on occasion the operating schedule has had to be cancelled on certain days because the blood supply was exhausted and the surgeons did not care to proceed without available supply. More restraint in the use of the Red Cross blood service has had to be requested.

Today the public recognizes the need for the availability of a good supply of blood. Donors take pride in giving their blood regularly. Red Cross blood donor lapel pins are worn with rightful pride.

In addition to its outpost and transfusion services the Society – or, more accurately, the Junior Red Cross – was responsible for establishing a few outstanding paediatric institutions. The Junior Red Cross Hospital for Crippled Children was begun in Calgary in 1922. It received substantial support from the Society over the years but it was becoming increasingly difficult to finance without sacrificing other valuable Red Cross programs. In 1956 it was turned over to voluntary community control. It has since become the Alberta Children's Hospital.

From 1924 to 1930 the Junior Red Cross operated a wing of the University Hospital in Edmonton for the care of handicapped children. A unit was set up in Regina in 1924 and operated until 1960 when it was transferred to the Regina General Hospital. The Junior Red Cross developed a convalescent unit at the Winnipeg Children's Hospital providing physical therapy facilities. It also provided a small unit in the hospital at Chateauguay, Quebec, and orthopaedic, dental and speech therapy clinics at various other locations.

Service Clubs and Foundations
A variety of other organizations besides the Grenfell Association and the Red Cross have contributed generously in establishing and maintaining hospital services. Service clubs such as the Shriners (which established two fine Hospitals for Crippled Children in Winnipeg and Montreal in the mid-twenties), the Rotarians, Kiwanians, and others have been active in providing services and facilities for hospital patients over the years.

Foundations have sponsored many innovations of direct interest and consequence to others. The millions spent by the Rockefeller Foundation, the Commonwealth Fund and others in support of medical education, nursing education and research have been mentioned already. In addition, much credit for the development of many aspects of education in the hospital, nursing and related fields in Canada must be given to the W.K. Kellogg Foundation of Battle Creek, Michigan.

The philanthropy of the Kellogg Foundation has been directed for many years by Dr Emory Morris, originally with Graham Davis in charge of the hospital division of its work. When Davis left the foundation in 1951 his mantle fell on the capable shoulders of Andrew Pattullo who has become the friend of worthy pioneer undertakings in the hospital field since that date. At the time of writing he was vice-president in charge of the foundation's programs.

The foundation has helped fund graduate courses in hospital administration at Toronto, Montreal, Alberta and Saskatchewan. It has given large sums to further undergraduate and graduate medical education at Dalhousie, British Columbia, Toronto, Sherbrooke and McMaster, and to the Association of Canadian Medical Colleges. It has contributed heavily to nursing education, supporting programs at the Universities of New Brunswick, Western Ontario, Toronto, McGill, Montreal and Saskatchewan and by the Canadian Nurses's Association. The Canadian Nurses' Foundation, set up in 1962 to provide bursaries and scholarships for nurses studying at the master's and doctoral levels and for grants to research in nursing service, received a $150,000 gift from the foundation. Considerable support has been given, also, to the dental field in Manitoba, to the Canadian Dental Association, and to dental education at universities, including Dalhousie, Toronto, McGill, and Montreal. Projects have been financed for the Canadian Hospital Association, the Canadian Education Association and the Associated Hospitals of Manitoba. Various universities including Queen's, Memorial, Laval and Ottawa, various associations and several government departments have received substantial support for fellowships and for loan and scholarship funds. Even individual hospitals have received help for unique and promising projects. To the end of 1970 the Kellogg Foundation had contributed to the hospital, nursing and medical fields in Canada amounts totalling more than $6.5 million.

In many ways some of the most valuable voluntary contributions have been those made within the hospital. Throughout the nineteenth century and on many occasions since then, individual citizens of a community have joined together to build, equip and maintain their hospital. Records show that many of the housekeeping and clerical duties of running the hospital were distributed among volunteers.

Within the hospital, doctors, nurses and other personnel have worked long hours and made great sacrifices in their personal lives in the interests of patient care. Trustees have devoted many hours and assumed heavy responsibilities without remuneration. With the exception of most doctors, hospital staffs have always served for less than competitive wages.

Hospital volunteers have helped thousands of patients over the years and made hospitals 'warmer' and in many ways more comfortable. The first women's auxiliary[12] appeared at the general hospital in St Catharines, Ontario, in 1865, and was known in that city for many years as the ladies' aid. This association and others proved so successful that women's auxiliaries spread to the majority of Canadian hospitals. At first concerned with such tasks as rolling bandages, sewing linens and fund raising, their activities have expanded gradually to include publicity and public relations, the operation of service carts and shops, and a multitude of other functions assisting patients and their relatives. The hospital administration has gradually assumed responsibility for the orientation and general direction of volunteers to ensure the most effective use of their services.

Beginning in 1910 in Ontario, auxiliaries have formed provincial associations (in all but one province) and in 1951 the Canadian Association of Women's Auxiliaries was organized with Mrs O.W. Rhynas of Ontario as the first president. Largely as a result of the work of these and related associations, auxiliary leaders have become better trained, more knowledgeable about the hospital and its role in the community.

12 Because of a small but increasing male membership, some auxiliaries are now known as 'hospital auxiliaries.'

Besides auxiliaries, other volunteers such as 'candy-stripers' and members of voluntary, disease-oriented societies provide an assortment of patient services.

As early as the 1840s some religious organizations were providing home care for the indigent sick. Other societies and organizations have carried on this Canadian tradition ever since.

Some of these agencies, such as the Health League of Canada (established in 1918) or the Victorian Order of Nurses (1897) have been primarily concerned with problems of public health; not until the past decade or two, during which time the scope of hospital activities has broadened to include more extensive ambulatory and home-care services, have their activities affected hospitals directly. Insofar as they improved or maintained the health of large numbers of people who might otherwise have become hospitalized, these agencies considerably relieved the pressure on hospital resources.

Other disease-oriented agencies such as the Canadian Mental Health Association, the Canadian Tuberculosis and Respiratory Disease Association, the Cancer Societies, the Heart Foundations, the Canadian Arthritis and Rheumatism Society and many others, have been formed to help plug gaps in the health delivery system. Besides funding research, pressuring government to face its responsibilities in the health field, and educating the public and health professionals, these voluntary agencies have provided numerous services for patients. Much of the agencies' work is carried on by volunteers.

The membership of most of the voluntary agencies is composed in large part of concerned doctors, nurses and other health workers, former patients and their relatives. In addition, there are many members who have not been touched so directly by health tragedy but who have been sensitive and concerned enough to spend a great deal of time and effort helping those in need.

THE ROLE OF THE PROVINCIAL AND FEDERAL GOVERNMENTS

Historically, Canadian hospitals have been founded and developed largely through the voluntary efforts of concerned individuals and groups. The provincial and federal governments, however, have also played important roles.

There are only a few specific references to health in the British North America Act. The Act assigns to the federal government the responsibilities for 'quarantine and the establishment and maintenance of marine hospitals.' To the provincial governments were assigned the powers related to 'the establishment, maintenance and management of hospitals, asylumns, charities and eleemosynary institutions in and for the provinces, other than marine hospitals.' Subsequent constitutional interpretations have placed responsibility for other health facilities and services predominantly with the provinces.

At first the provinces largely restricted their activities to sporadic assistance to municipalities in setting up ad hoc (and then permanent) boards of health and to the building and maintenance of mental institutions. The 1875 Public Health Act in the United Kingdon which assigned to municipalities the responsibility for setting up boards of health had a marked effect in Canada. Every province – beginning with Ontario in 1884 – passed legislation based on the British act. The early local boards of health were primarily concerned with environmental sanitation and communicable diseases. By 1920, programs promoting maternal and child health care, general health education and personal health supervision were well under way.

Concerned with providing medical assistance to the poor and financial assistance to hospitals treating them, some provinces began per diem grants and enacted laws requiring municipalities to bear hospitalization costs of their indigent residents. Most of the early legislation affecting hospitals was concerned with safeguarding government grants. Inspectors were appointed to visit the hospitals and check the registers to ensure that the regulations were not being abused. The provincial governments were concerned with building codes and geographical distribution of hospitals. Not until the 1930s and 1940s was any legislative interest shown in the internal procedures of the hospital.

To administer these public health and hospital regulations, some provinces set up a board of health or its equivalent. In other areas responsibilities were distributed among such departments as agriculture, municipal affairs, natural resources and the provincial secretary.

The first department of health in Canada was established in New Brunswick in 1918. Dr W.F. Roberts, later president of the Canadian Public Health Association, was the first minister. The other provinces formed separate departments with jurisdiction solely over health (or occasionally health and welfare) in the following order: Alberta (1919), Saskatchewan and Ontario (1923), Manitoba (1928), Nova Scotia and Prince Edward Island (1931), Quebec (1936) and British Columbia (1946). Newfoundland formed a department of health and welfare in 1934 before the island joined Confederation.

Most health functions are exercised directly by the departments of health. But some programs in some provinces have been assigned to semi-independent boards or commissions directly responsible to the minister of health. This has often resulted when a province has moved into an area previously administered by a voluntary agency or when it has beeen deemed advisable 'to keep the politics out' of a program. For example, tuberculosis services, hospital and medical insurance, cancer control and alcoholism programs have sometimes been administered by government agencies.

Many provinces have taken over direct sponsorship of public health and hospital-service programs combatting communicable diseases (such as tuberculosis and venereal diseases), cancer and crippling disabilities. Other services provided by provincial (or local) health organizations have come to include provincial laboratories, public health nursing and the provision of detailed data, information and advice through statistical and consultant services.

The provinces have helped to improve hospital standards by authorizing registration bodies for the licensing of health-care personnel and by sponsoring improved educational services and research demonstration projects. Provincial subsidization of health services in remote and poverty-stricken areas has helped to alleviate regional disparities in the availability and quality of health care.

Provincial governments have worked closely with – and often subsidized – voluntary health agencies especially in promoting education, both lay and professional.

Without doubt the provincial hospital and medical insurance plans have had the greatest effect on hospitals. Over the years, governments had become increasingly concerned about the inability of growing numbers of patients to pay their health costs. This concern extended to the subsequent financial difficulties of hospitals. The more that governments have contributed, the more they have become determined to ensure that their funds are well spent. With 30 percent more of the provincial budget going to health services – and most of that to hospital care – provincial controls have become stringent.[13]

With notable exceptions in Quebec and Nova Scotia, provincial governments have been responsible generally for building and operating mental

13 See Chapter 5.

institutions. In some cases, tuberculosis sanatoria have come under greater provincial sponsorship and direction. Rarely, however, have the provinces owned and operated active treatment hospitals. For many years the Victoria General in Halifax and the University of Alberta Hospital in Edmonton were the only exceptions outside Newfoundland.

Despite the outstanding efforts of the Grenfell Association and other voluntary groups there were still many outports in that island colony without medical and hospital services. During the depression, the government had become insolvent and was superceded by a Commission of Government which among other acts initiated a system of cottage hospitals. Starting at Old Perlican on the east shore, fourteen small hospitals were built before the island joined Confederation in 1949. (Three more were opened later.) They ranged in size from eight beds (Fogo) to thirty-two beds (Come-by-Chance) but averaged about twenty. The staff usually consisted of a doctor, frequently a British FRCS, two graduate nurses, three to five ward aides, frequently a laboratory technologist, domestic staff, a janitor-orderly and a hospital secretary who administered the local prepayment health insurance plan for the hospital district.

Some years ago, I visited these outport hospitals by aircraft and boat. The road connections to these isolated villages were, at that time, poor or non-existent. The quality and quantity of the work done was impressive, especially in view of the major difficulties encountered. Several hospitals generated their own electricity. Almost all lacked what we would consider today to be essential equipment; some sterilized instruments at atmospheric pressure because no autoclave was available. Sometimes one nurse had to handle a confinement while the doctor operated. This meant that the other nurse acted as anaesthetist while the ward aide served as surgical assistant. Nurses learned other emergency surgical and medical procedures for the occasions when bad weather stranded the doctor at a distance from the hospital.

By the late sixties medical staff in each of the cottage hospitals had increased and there remained but a few where only a single physician was on staff. Many of the physicians, however, engaged in private practice and spent only a portion of their time in the hospital. Facilities in virtually all of the outport hospitals now include diagnostic X-ray equipment and a modern laboratory as well as operating and delivery rooms. Not surprisingly the community and district public health programs are hospital based.

Although more than twenty hospitals are owned by the government, potential problems of bureaucratic delays and inflexible regulations have been largely avoided by judicious delegation of authority to hospital administrative and medical staff. The officials in the Newfoundland Department of Health during the early 1950s – and those who have served since – were hard working, competent and dedicated. During those early years of the Newfoundland outport hospitals (and probably continuing today although I do not have personal knowledge to back this assumption), everyone on the hospital staff sensed a direct responsibility to the patient. I believe it was the *lack* of governmental bureaucracy which inspired this devotion; it was not uncommon to see government hospital officials visit outport hospitals and personally comfort individuals who were ill.

Over the fifty years surveyed in this book, the role of the federal government in the operation of hospitals and health care has expanded dramatically. As we have seen, the BNA Act conferred on Ottawa the responsibility for quarantine services and medical treatment for ailing seamen. In time, however, these responsibilities grew to include health care for active members of the armed services and some limited care for the Indian and Eskimo peoples. At the conclusion of the first world war the federal government was faced with the duty to build and maintain hospitals for a large number of wounded veterans, all entitled to government care.

The Department of Health, as it was first called, was established in 1919. The department brought together the medical and quarantine services of the Department of Immigration and Colonization, the marine hospital service from Marine and Fisheries, the food and drug laboratories from Trade and Commerce and other similar services. A publicity and statistics division was created; venereal disease and child welfare divisions were initiated; hygiene laboratories were funded.

The new Dominion Council of Health included the chief medical officer (later deputy minister) of each provincial department or board of health, the deputy minister of the federal government plus five other persons appointed by the governor-general-in-council to represent various sectors of society. A scientific advisor for public health was also appointed. This Dominion Council of Health has met twice yearly in Ottawa and has fulfilled a valuable role in facilitating the exchange of information, integrating services and developing recommended policies.

In 1928 the Department of Health merged with the Department of Soldiers' Civil Re-establishment to become the Department of Pensions and National Health. In 1944 it was re-named the Department of National Health and Welfare, with a deputy minister to administer each of its two divisions.

All of the federal department's activities have had some effect – even an indirect effect – on hospitals. Some of the increased activity has had momentous impact. The federal government has provided huge grants to stimulate the expansion of hospitals and to help improve health teaching facilities. In co-operation with the provincial governments, Ottawa inaugurated a national, prepaid hospital plan and later a similar plan covering medical services. Finally, the federal department undertook to provide direct medical service to the Indians and Eskimos.

The provision of public health and treatment programs for Canada's indigenous people was totally inadequate before the second world war. Conflicts over jurisdictional responsibility, lack of money and personnel retarded progress. Most of all, lack of concern and interest created a vacuum. The first hospital built specifically for Indians was at Norway House, Manitoba. Others followed during the twenties and thirties at Gleichen, Cardston, Brocket and Morley in Alberta; Oshweken, Ontario; Fort Qu'Appelle, Saskatchewan and four or five other places, mostly in Manitoba. In 1945 the Charles Camsell Hospital was built in Edmonton and has continuously provided a very high standard of medical care. Only in 1945 did the newly created Department of National Health and Welfare assume full responsibility for Indian health services.

From about twenty hospitals and nursing stations in 1946, the department expanded its services during the next decade so that by 1957 some eighteen hospitals and about forty nursing stations were in operation. A great deal of credit must go to Dr Percy E. Moore, who directed and greatly improved Indian health services from 1939 to 1965.

In the early years the primary concern was tuberculosis. While still serious, this disease is slowly being brought under control. However, the health standards of the indigenous peoples are still far below Canadian averages.

The federal government has long held jurisdictional responsibility for ensuring the co-ordination of health care for all residents of the Northwest Territories and the Yukon. However, not until the late 1950s did it meet this responsibility by building and operating hospitals. To be sure, there were nine or ten nursing stations built in the far north by the federal government during the period 1945 to 1957. Most of the hospitals, however, were built and run under religious auspices.

In 1954 the Department of National Health and Welfare expanded the old Indian Health Services Directorate to include Northern Health Services. Assuming direct control of a couple of hospitals previously operated by the Yukon Territorial Government and building elsewhere, this new Directorate, which was later (1962) incorporated into a Medical Services Branch, acted in many ways as a department of health to the territorial councils.

To overcome problems of distance, transportation and communication, air service has been used increasingly during the sixties to facilitate medical relief. A vigorous recruiting program has been inaugurated to attract competent professionals, many of whom require special training. In more recent years efforts have begun to train greater numbers of permanent residents in the health professions.

In 1970 the Medical Service Branch operated fourteen hospitals, including five in the northern territories, in co-operation with other community and mission facilities. In remote areas the branch supports some fifty-seven nursing stations which are staffed by one or two nurses providing emergency treatment and public health services. There are also numerous health centres and health stations with out-patient clinics and other health programs.

Although federal government health services continue to expand in the northern territories, it has been the objective of the Department of National Health and Welfare since the mid-sixties to integrate the health services now reserved for Indians and Eskimos into the provincial and local health services.

Before the first world war, the federal government had cared for its active militiamen and disabled veterans in civilian hospitals. By 1915, however, the mounting causualty lists put a strain on the arrangement and Ottawa created the Military Hospitals Commission. At first the commission sought to place wounded veterans in private homes but this arrangement was inadequate in both the quantity of beds available and the quality of medical care.

In 1917 the government authorized the commission to start on an intensive program of hospital building. By the spring of 1920 the commission[14] had built or renovated forty-four hospitals providing active treatment, convalescent, domiciliary, psychiatric and tuberculosis care and a variety of outpatient and rehabilitative services. At the same time there were more than fifty civilian hospitals with which the department had negotiated agreements for the provision of treatment for veterans.

The number of veterans requiring hospitalization declined during the mid and late 1920s and those who did need hospital care were most often afflicted with a disability of a chronic nature. By 1928 (when the Departments of Health and of Soldiers' Civil Re-establishment were merged to form the Department of Pensions and National Health) there were fewer than 2,500 veterans under treatment. During the thirties the guiding spirit

14 By this time the commission had been re-named the Invalided Soldiers' Commission in the Department of Soldiers' Civil Re-establishment.

of veteran rehabilitation was Dr Ross Millar, formerly a physician from Amherst, Nova Scotia. His zealous interest in the welfare of the veteran was appreciated from coast to coast; his delight in achieving construction economies was gladly shared with all within earshot. Did he not build the Veterans' Building at the Ottawa Civic Hospital for $700 a bed? 'Now you fellows match that,' he would bellow so that the entire floor could hear.

During the second world war, a similar pattern emerged with an intensive building program followed by a gradually decreasing case load. The maximum number of veterans' beds in DVA institutions and other hospitals was 12,118 in 1946.

From the time of their establishment during the first world war, the Canadian military hospitals were staffed with doctors employed as civil servants. At first, this condition of employment posed no particular problems, but by the end of the second world war certain disadvantages were beginning to be manifest.

For one thing, the aging veterans from the first world war who were still hospitalized suffered more from the normal disorders of the elderly than from the wounds which put them in the hospital in the first place. The civil-service physicians found they were less experienced in geriatric cases than the physician in private practice whose case load is drawn from the public at large. In addition, the veterans' hospitals had no connection with university medical schools. Such a connection is always an advantage, but in the large and complex institutions that most DVA hospitals had become, its lack was a massive disadvantage.

For these and other reasons, the newly formed Department of Veterans' Affairs instituted in 1945 a policy of granting some hospital privileges to physicians not employed as civil servants. Under the leadership of Dr William Warner, ably advised by Dr Duncan Graham, under whom he had trained, the former defects were recognized and the federal government began to normalize and improve the situation.

Many veterans' hospitals started post-graduate programs in a variety of specialties with the help and approval of the RCPS(C). This also ensured the best possible care for veterans. Although some of the early institutions were hastily designed and built under wartime emergency conditions, they soon came to provide a superior quality of care and many won full accreditation for their services. As time went on and the patronage of veterans diminished, some of the DVA hospitals began to accept other patients, requiring only that their medical care would be directed by the members of the hospital staff.

Then, to further integrate the treatment of veterans with civilian care, certain veterans were no longer required to receive treatment in DVA or approved hospitals. Rather they were authorized to choose their own doctor and hospital, an arrangement considerably more convenient for those living in communities some distance removed from the veterans' hospitals.

By the early 1960s the department was seriously questioning the necessity to continue the operation of a chain of well-equipped hospitals across Canada at considerable expense when the essential services to veterans could be provided elsewhere at less cost. Dr Kenneth Ritchie, director of hospital services of the Department of Veterans' Affairs, has stated on numerous occasions that the department is not primarily in the business of operating hospitals and is willing to turn these facilities over to responsible bodies provided there could be continuing assurance that the veterans would be cared for and that there would always be available a stipulated number of beds for their care.

In 1963 the Department of Veterans' Affairs announced this policy of transferring control of veterans' hospitals to universities and other bodies wherever possible. This was the result of a desire to maintain the university affiliation and teaching programs of the veterans' hospitals, yet at the same time avoid the cost of having a growing number of vacancies resulting from the decrease in active treatment cases and the demise of many older veterans residing in hospital as chronic and domiciliary patients. Since then, Sunnybrook Hospital in Toronto has been transferred to the University of Toronto and l'Hôpital Ste Foy in Quebec City has been transferred to Laval University.

In 1970 the Department of Veterans' Affairs continued to operate nine hospitals in Canada.

3
Hospital associations

Many years ago hospitals were simple institutions with few financial and administrative problems. They had minimal or no contact with government, professional associations or even with each other. As hospitals grew into increasingly complex centres for medical care, new problems developed – problems which hospitals could not deal with satisfactorily as individual institutions.

To help solve these problems and generally to improve many facets of hospital performance, hospital associations have been formed. These bodies have served primarily as educational media whereby hospital personnel have exchanged ideas and become better informed. Conventions, publications, conferences, workshops, library services and extension courses have all contributed.

Hospital associations have represented hospitals collectively in dealing not only with governments but with professional associations, allied health organizations and the general public. These contacts have always been important and crucially so in the past decade or two as hospital operating and construction costs have risen drastically, the hospital has increasingly evolved toward a community health centre and regional planning has become imperative.

Hospital associations have always served society indirectly through their services to hospitals. They have also provided various direct services including the establishment and operation of non-profit Blue Cross hospital insurance plans.

It is of interest that the provincial and national hospital bodies in Canada have had a large proportion of trustees among their presidents and senior officers. Looking back over the years and thinking of the many trustees who have sat on association boards, one is impressed by the tremendous aggregate contribution which these men and women have made to hospital progress, a contribution all the more impressive when we realize that most of these trustees not only served without remuneration but at considerable personal sacrifice because of reduced concentration of their own livelihood.

Not the least of the benefits associated with trustee leadership has been the influence wielded by these men and women in getting legislative support for highly desirable measures and regulations. In such matters as improved financial support for hospitals and in the development of a workable transition from voluntary hospital insurance to provincially sponsored plans, the political and community stature of many of these altruistic citizens who spoke for the hospitals has been of inestimable value.

Needless to say, administrators and other hospital personnel have also served with remarkable devotion. Through all of their efforts hospital associations in Canada have made considerable contributions to hospital efficiency and standards of patient care.

THE ORIGINAL CANADIAN HOSPITAL ASSOCIATION

The first hospital association in Canada seems to have been a short-lived organization called the Ontario Hospital Association. From its name one would judge that its intentions were limited to a provincial scale. And from the records available it met twice only – once at its founding meeting and again in 1904, apparently its last meeting.

The first attempt to organize a national hospital association was made in 1907. Dr J.N.E. Brown, the energetic superintendent of the old Toronto General Hospital on Gerrard Street East, was soliciting membership in the eight-year-old American Medical Association.[1] Canadian interest in the AHA was high and Dr Brown concluded that an association of Canadian hospital superintendents was not only possible but desirable. In the spring of 1907 his work paid off and the original Canadian Hospital Association was formed at Toronto. Although this organization pre-dated the half century under consideration, I include an account of its beginnings for historical perspective.

1 In its earliest years this organization had been known as the Hospital Association of the United States and Canada.

At the first meeting in the Ontario Parliament Buildings, the superintendents of forty-nine hospitals were present. Among them were Dr Donald M. Robertson of the Protestant General Hospital, Ottawa (later of the Ottawa Civic Hospital); Miss M.A. Snively, superintendent of the Nurses Training School, Toronto General Hospital; Dr B.E. Mackenzie of the Orthopaedic Hospital, Toronto (now part of Toronto East General Hospital); Dr John Ferguson, chief of medicine at the Toronto Western Hospital; Dr C.K. Clarke, head of the Asylum for the Insane on Queen Street in Toronto, and for some years superintendent of the Toronto General Hospital and dean of the University of Toronto Faculty of Medicine; and Dr Edward Ryan of Rockwood Hospital (Mental), Kingston, Ontario. Limited to superintendents and their assistants at first, the association broadened its membership to include trustees in 1908.

Speakers at the first meeting included Dr Helen MacMurchy, concerned at this early time with public health measures related to new mothers and their infants, and Dr John A. Amyot, then provincial bacteriologist in Ontario and later deputy minister of national health. Dr Renwick R. Ross of Buffalo, NY, president of the American Hospital Association, also gave an address, as did Dr R. Bruce Smith, Inspector of Hospitals for Ontario, long a key hospital figure in that province. The Honorable J.J. Foy, Ontario attorney-general, and the Honorable J.W. Hanna, provincial secretary, also attended.

I remember the government figures well as I was a page boy in the Ontario Legislature at that time. Memory fails me – I cannot remember if I listened in on the founding meeting of the original CHA or not. It's quite possible I did for we were curious young lads, interested in the proceedings whether governmental or otherwise.

Although this meeting was called to set up a national association, the delegates, a few visitors excepted, were all Ontario hospital administrators. At this late date it is impossible to assess the founders' intent but it seems likely that the use of the broader name must have been a move to start with a local nucleus and then expand to a wider base of membership. Three of the eight members of the executive committee of the association were from Quebec, Nova Scotia and Manitoba, reflecting an effort to make this a national body right from the start.

This early association was concerned with broadening its membership, not only geographically, but to include trustees and nurses. Various attempts were made to amalgamate the CHA with the Association of Superintendents of Training Schools and the Graduate Nurses Association. To this end a joint meeting was held in Niagara Falls in 1911. In the same year a CHA committee was set up 'to consider and arrange a constitution as a working basis for some national organization.'

The presidents of the original Canadian Hospital Association were:

1907–08 Miss Louise Brent, Toronto
1908–09 Dr W.J. Dobbie, Toronto
1909–10 H.E. Webster, Montreal
1910–11 Miss C.F. Green, Belleville, Ontario
1911–13 Dr H.A. Boyce, Kingston, Ontario
1913   Dr E.H. Young, Kingston, Ontario

The first meeting of the CHA did little more than establish the organization and arrange to have annual meetings. It did, however, invite the American Hospital Association to meet in Toronto in 1908 and the AHA did convene for the first time in Canada under the presidency of Dr S.S. Goldwater, the distinguished administrator of Mount Sinai Hospital in New York, and with J. Ross Robertson of Toronto, historian, newspaper publisher and chairman of the board of the Hospital for Sick Children, as senior vice-president. Oddly enough, the AHA and the CHA did not meet at the same time.

About 1910 the CHA began to broaden its functions and services. Committees were set up to establish a uniform, efficient accounting system for small hospitals and to petition the federal government to revise the tariff on various hospital supplies.

A hospital journal, *Hospital World*, was published in Toronto by Dr G.A. Young whom I remember as a striking figure of a man with silver hair, a well-spiked mustache, a compelling personality and the brightest of yellow gloves. His journal became the official organ of the CHA in 1912. As a reflection of its increased activities, membership fees in the CHA rose from one to two dollars in 1910 and to three dollars in 1913.

The annual meeting for 1914 was scheduled for Toronto in October but the outbreak of war intervened. Association activities were suspended until the cessation of hostilities – and were never revived. That the association was not resurrected was not Dr G.A. Young's fault. When the Armistice was signed in 1918 he insisted editorially in *Hospital World* that the officers of the CHA were shirking their responsibilities by not calling annual meetings. *Hospital World* still proclaimed itself the offical organ of the Canadian Hospital Association until 1920. But Dr Young's yellow gloves were ineffectual, so he changed his magazine's title to *Hospital, Medical and Nursing World* and it became the official journal of 'the provincial hospital associations,' specifically, those of British Columbia and Alberta.

The last record of the CHA which I have been able to find was in the minutes of the organizational meeting of the Ontario Hospital Association in 1923. It was noted there that Dr W.J. Dobbie was secretary of the CHA, having assumed that position when Dr J.N.E. Brown moved to Detroit in 1913. The record did not indicate any CHA activity after 1914.

THE CANADIAN HOSPITAL COUNCIL (ASSOCIATION)

In order to better appreciate the origins of the ambitious series of programs which culminated in the creation of a Department of Hospital Service and ultimately the Canadian Hospital Council, one should begin with the 1921 annual meeting of the Canadian Medical Association.

The hospitals of this country have been deeply indebted to the CMA. Without its leadership in many undertakings affecting hospitals, the improvement in our hospital system would have been greatly delayed.

Following the first world war the Canadian Medical Association was in a desperate situation. Although more than fifty years old by this time, the association was perennially afflicted with difficulties in persuading potential members of the desirability of a national medical organization. The war had hindered CMA programs and services within Canada and by 1921 its financial position was so bad that dissolution seemed imminent. Even the president, Dr Murdock Chisholm, was pessimistic.

It is largely to the credit of the doughty Dr John McEachern of Calgary that the association did not fold up. This slow-spoken pipe smoker with the determined chin would not admit defeat. At the Halifax meeting of the CMA in 1921 he drafted courses of action for the national and provincial medical bodies; and by initiating a bond issue to which the doctors freely subscribed, he paved the way for a remarkable financial rejuvenation of the CMA.

This 1921 annual meeting was a milestone for other reasons. Aware of the distrust of many doctors of the new American College of Surgeons' standardization requirements, the CMA passed a resolution expressing 'unqualified approval of the plan of standardization of the hospitals of the Dominion as being now undertaken under the supervision of Dr M.T. MacEachern of Vancouver.'

In addition, the decision to appoint Dr T.C. Routley[2] as a full-time secretary with suitable remuneration 'when funds permitted' assured the association of many years of progressive leadership. Under his direction and with the help of many others, the CMA never looked back. Dr Routley's management of the broadening scope of activities earned for him the deep

2 Dr Routley was associate secretary until 1923, when he became general secretary.

respect and admiration of hospital and medical men across the continent and eventually in many other lands.

Dr Routley had been christened Thomas Clarence and it was a curiosity to me during the many years of our association in the CMA secretariat that he was known in western Canada as Tom and as Clarence in the east. From 1928 to 1945 I was privileged to serve him as associate secretary of the CMA. Perhaps his greatest ability was in reconciling conflicting viewpoints. Time and again I watched and listened at board-table discussions as he would hear out regional representatives. Then, quietly and modestly, he would ask the chairman's permission to sum up the debate. From one man's argument he would pick out a point, re-word it slightly and the man's head would nod vigorously in approval. Then he would re-word another point and another; two more heads would nod agreement. Then he would propose a resolution which encompassed bits and pieces of every suggestion made; he would be barely finished with this exercise when the motion was moved, seconded and adopted.

Clarence Routley was an accomplished amateur pianist. On at least one occasion I saw him put this ability to good use for the CMA. I accompanied him to a regional meeting in a Prairie town where the local doctors had sworn to tear him and the CMA apart on some contentious issue now long since forgotten. Dr Routley's preparation for the possibly stormy meeting was simple; he wired ahead asking that a piano be installed in the meeting hall and that a local physician with a fine tenor voice be in attendance.

Dr Routley and his singing companion arrived early and started a round of old standard songs. As each new arrival entered the hall he gravitated to the singing group and soon found himself bellowing out the old favorites. When the chairman finally called the meeting to order, the animosities had been forgotten, mountainous grievances had been reduced to molehills and the meeting glided to an early conclusion.

In the early 1930s, the CMA faced a crisis when the famed Mayo Clinic of Rochester, Minnesota, offered Dr Routley the job of general director at a fabulous salary. He must have been tempted and flattered – any mortal would have been – but he eventually turned the offer down. He preferred to stay in Canada (his ancestors had been United Empire Loyalists) and continue his work with the CMA. In turn, the CMA showed its appreciation by increasing Dr Routley's salary as general secretary.

Dr Routley was a major figure in the formation of the World Medical Association in 1947 in Paris. He was elected the chairman of the WMA's General Council and in 1950 headed a WMA group which toured the world studying medical needs in many countries.

The term 'disorganized medicine' might be more appropriately applied to the condition of our affairs when T.C.R. took over [wrote his successor, A.D. Kelly, in the *Canadian Medical Association Journal* in 1959] but through hard work, infectious enthusiasm and shrewd business sense oddly combined with the missionary spirit, he wrought a miracle. To him, more than to any other individual, we owe the progress which the Association made during the thirty-one years in which he added lustre to the post of General Secretary.'

Following Dr Routley's appointment as the CMA's general secretary, the association launched a vigorous program to encourage postgraduate medical education. After receiving presentations by Drs A.T. Bazin and C.C. Birchard of Montreal, the Sun Life Assurance of Canada agreed to finance postgraduate tours across the country by leading medical educators. A team of eastern doctors toured the west and a team of westerners went east, holding intensive one-day sessions for doctors in centres in the various provinces. The trips, sometimes lasting as long as three weeks, were often exhausting. However the programs were tremendously successful and were worth the effort. This happy arrangement continued until the depression dismantled the program in 1932. During its operation Sun Life contributed some $212,000 to this educational program beamed primarily at doctors in smaller communities.

In 1927, B.T. Macaulay, president of Sun Life, was so pleased with the use of these funds that he asked Dr Routley to suggest another worthy project.

The most obvious need was to improve hospital standards across the country. The Council of the Canadian Medical Association, at its 1926 meeting in Victoria, set up a Committee on Hospital Efficiency under the chairmanship of Dr Malcolm R. Bow of Regina, later a key figure in the Alberta Department of Health. A conference on hospital efficienty was held with addresses by the Honorable James H. King, federal minister of health; Dr F.N.G. Starr of Toronto, president-elect of the CMA; Dr Alexander Primrose of Toronto; Dr John A. Amyot, deputy minister of health for Canada; Dr H.H. Murphy of Kamloops; Dr Alphonse Lessard of Quebec; Dr G. Stewart Cameron of Peterborough, Ontario; Dr George A. Ramsay of London, Ontario; Dr Grant Fleming of Montreal; Dr J.C. Meakins of Montreal; and Dr James Miller of Kingston, Ontario. Dr S.E. Moore of Regina outlined how the organization could be effective, first on the provincial level, and then on a national basis. He detailed its functions and how it could be financed.

In 1927 the CMA formally approved setting up a Department of Hospital Service which the Sun Life Assurance Company of Canada agreed to support financially. A small committee was named to work out a program of direction for the new department. A committee composed of Drs J.G. Fitzgerald, director of the University of Toronto's School of Hygiene, Harvey Smith of Winnipeg, G.S. Cameron of Peterborough, F.W. Routley (brother of T.C. Routley) of the Canadian Red Cross, A.T. Bazin of Montreal, Duncan Graham of Toronto, J.G. MacDougall of Halifax, and H.H. Murphy of Kamloops, met and advised setting up an Advisory Committee to the Department, composed of Drs A.K. Haywood, Montreal (chairman); L.A. Lessard, Montreal; F.W. Routley, Toronto; George F. Stephens, Winnipeg; H.R. Smith, Edmonton; and Frederick C. Bell, Vancouver. The recommendation was accepted and approved.

Choosing Alf Haywood as chairman was a stroke of genius. He loved people and, even more so, loved to do something for them. While at the Montreal General Hospital, he was always helping some other hospital – advising, sending over an expert in something-or-other, or giving somebody else's staff personnel an intensive refresher course on one of his services. (It was for being helpful to others during the first world war that he received an OBE.) He was largely instrumental in getting the Montreal Hospital Council set up in 1926, the first organization bringing together the French- and English-speaking superintendents and board chairmen. He was delightfully frank; he could tear a man to pieces (including myself) and immediately work out for him a new approach to his problem. At one convention, after he had accepted the post at the Vancouver General Hospital during one of those invaluable evening 'bull sessions' in somebody's room when the day's paper are *really* dissected, Alf disagreed vehemently with his chairman, an equally frank and devastating labor leader, James H. McVety, who was never at a loss for the right phrase. Their eloquence would have commanded respect from a veteran sergeant-major.

Haywood's proudest boast was that three of his 'boys' became president of the American Hospital Association – Dr Donald C. Smelzer of Lankenau Hospital, Philadelphia; Dr Basil C. MacLean of Strong Memorial Hospital, Rochester, later Hospital Commissioner of New York City; and Dr Peter Ward of Charles T. Miller Hospital, St Paul, Minnesota. No other senior administrator has ever equalled that record. He himself was once offered the official nomination for the AHA presidency but declined, feeling that the Vancouver General Hospital needed his full attention at that time.

When the CMA set up its Department of Hospital Service in January, 1928, it was my good fortune that Dr Haywood was made chairman of the Hospital Advisory Committee. Nothing was too much trouble. He spent days with me at his own hospital, then the Montreal General, going over the problems of hospitals and discussing the endless developments that were needed in the field.

To administer the new department, the CMA created the post of associate secretary. I was offered the appointment and making the decision to take it or not was one of the most difficult of my life. At the time I was assistant to Dr F. Arnold Clarkson, chief of medicine at Toronto Western Hospital. The work was exciting, a daily challenge, and the experience was heightened by working for Dr Clarkson, a physician of piercing intelligence and wit. Additionally I was teaching clinical medicine to the final-year medical students from the University of Toronto. As a teacher my work was supervised by Professor Duncan A. Graham, head of medicine at the university. Working for Professor Graham was not always easy, but it was stimulating and a learning experience beyond compare; his dedicated insistence upon the maintenance of the highest standards in everything we did was a lifetime inspiration to his teachers and students alike.

So, I was happy in my work but intrigued with the CMA's offer of a position in which I would be able to treat 'sick hospitals'; I had seen a number of them on the Sun Life tours and I was impressed with the challenge. After consultation with some of my clinical colleagues, I resolved my doubts and decided to take the post.

The function of the Department of Hospital Service was to assist hospitals in every way possible – by maintaining a clearing-house for hospital information, by establishing a library service to hospital administrators, by making personal visits of consultation and advice, by furthering the establishment of provincial and regional hospital associations. From its inception, the services of the department were in great demand. The Canadian Hospital Council was set up. Provincial associations were assisted. The first hospital directory was compiled. A basis for approving hospitals for internship was developed and an approval committee set up. Standards for schools teaching laboratory technologists were worked out and an approval committee formed. Hospital plans were checked on request and planning advice given.

The enthusiastic reception granted the new department was gratifying, but, as I was soon to discover, the enthusiasm was sometimes accorded for misguided reasons.

On my first western tour in the new post I found that a number of prominent western doctors wholeheartedly endorsed the Department of Hospital Service primarily as a protest against the American College of Surgeons' accreditation-standardization program discussed earlier. They saw in the department the means by which the ACS program could 'be kicked out of Canada.'

I was stunned with this reaction; I had accepted the ACS program as excellent and, without knowing him personally, admired Dr 'Mac' MacEachern, the Canadian physician who administered it. I decided I should learn at first hand more about the program and the man who ran it. I spent a week in Chicago studying the ACS program and talking with Dr MacEachern. I returned to Canada convinced that the program – albeit one originating with an 'outside' organization – was the best thing that had ever happened to Canadian hospitals. Moreover, I returned with the conviction that rather than 'kick' Dr MacEachern out of his native country, we should give his program every assistance. Some day we would set up our own evaluation program but, for some years to come, we thought we could accomplish much more by working jointly on a common program. The executive committee of the Canadian Medical Association supported my viewpoint unanimously.

This was a fortunate decision; we in Canada benefited tremendously by our close relationship with this program and with its director who seemed to be at the centre of so many of the worthwhile developments in the hospital field.

Although the new Department of Hospital Service was fulfilling its intended function, it was not truly representative of the hospitals themselves – that is, of hospital management. Hospital administrators felt, with some logic, that their presentations to Ottawa, for instance, might carry more weight if put forward by the hospitals rather than at second hand through the department.

I had discussed these and related problems a number of times with Dr Fred W. Routley who was the Ontario director of the Red Cross and the founding secretary of the rapidly-growing Ontario Hospital Association. Dr Routley and I agreed on the need for an organization to more fully represent hospital management and we suggested that it be sponsored by the CMA through the Department of Hospital Service. The departmental committee and executive committee of the CMA approved the suggestion in 1931.

In September, 1931, the American Hospital Association was to hold its annual convention in Toronto; a Canadian doctor, George R. Stephens, director of the Winnipeg General Hospital, was to be installed as the AHA president at the convention. It seemed a logical time to bring up the question of a Canadian hospital organization, roughly comparable to the AHA model. Provincial and regional hospital associations were asked to attend the convention and contribute to a discussion of how to organize a national association.

The meeting agreed unanimously on the need for a national organization. But recognizing the need for something and achieving a means to meet the need are different things. 'How was the organization to be financed?' was one question which dogged the discussions. The Department of Hospital Service agreed to provide office and secretarial help for the few years needed to put the association on its financial feet. (As mentioned earlier, the department was in turn financed by Sun Life.)

An even trickier question concerned what *kind* of organization the hospitals wanted. For example, it was easy to see that with the extremely long distances to be travelled in Canada, an organization with personal – as opposed to institutional – membership would likely fail. Nor would it be practical – for sometime to come – to attempt to compete with the AHA's annual convention; the AHA meeting attracted many Canadian hospital administrators and was so 'packed with goodies' for those who attended that few doubted that the Canadian equivalent would fail miserably. (It was also true that, back in 1931, few Canadians – whether doctors or lay administrators – had acquired the taste for attending more than one convention per year.) These vexing problems were settled: membership was open to provincial or regional hospital associations and to the CMA through the Department of Hospital Service. The federal department of Pensions and National Health and the provincial departments of health were also eligible for membership; but to avoid embarrassment if the new organization decided to criticise the government or ask for financial help, the governmental representatives were to be non-voting members.

Finally, it seemed logical to name the new organization a 'council' rather than 'association.' The name carried a less formal connotation, and indicated a group of regional or provincial members who could be called into conference readily without all the attendant trappings of a national convention.

And so was born the Canadian Hospital Council (CHC).

My description of the council's emergence has been necessarily brief and only hints at some of the birth pains. There were others. Now, as I look back through my correspondence of the time, I recall that many administrators and board members did not view the new council with favor. The essential problem, as they saw it, was that their own local concerns would be submerged in a large, national body. They agreed on the need for provincial hospital associations; within those bodies, they believed, their local problems could be aired to an understanding and sympathetic audience. But a large, national organization would simply swamp the needs and requests of local hospitals.

This attitude has always been a problem in Canada in many fields of endeavor, not the hospital field alone. Too many of us know more about the problems of the states to our south than we do about the problems of our neighboring provinces.

Still, the council survived these quibblings and at its founding meeting at Toronto's Royal York Hotel there were twenty-six delegates and thirteen observers in attendance. (A complete list of those in attendance is contained in Appendix D.) Dr Fred W. Routley was elected the first president.

Frederick Routley was a physician, first and foremost, but for a man of such boundless enthusiasm, one career seemed hardly enough. As a young practitioner in the rural community of Maple, north of Toronto, he was fascinated with the telephone as a means of quick communication with patients. On his own he developed a regional telephone service. He became actively involved with the Red Cross and by 1922 was named as Ontario director. In that capacity he was impressed with the need for better hospitals and in 1923 organized the Ontario Hospital Association to further that end. The OHA's first convention was held in 1924 and it has not stopped growing since. For many years the association's 'office' was a filing cabinet in Dr Routley's Red Cross office. He was a strong supporter of the Canadian Hospital Council and it was entirely fitting that he was chosen its first president.

At its first meeting the Canadian Hospital Council arranged to meet every two years for a two-day session. One of its first actions was to prepare a brief to the federal government requesting tariff and excise concessions for public hospitals.

The Advisory Board on Tariff and Taxation, set up in 1926 (under the chairmanship of W.H. Moore, MP), had been holding public sessions. For some time the Department of Hospital Service of the CMA had been recommending to the board that public hospitals be permitted to import free of duty such equipment as operating tables, operating room lights, pressure sterilizers, special laboratory equipment and other articles essential to hospitals but not manufactured in Canada. Such import charges were not protective of Canadian industry and a tariff item productive only of revenue was not justified in the case of public hospitals already carrying a heavy burden of non-remunerative work. Hector B. McKinnon, secretary to the advisory board and later commissioner of tariffs in the Department of Finance, was most helpful in discussing the department's presentation and possible changes. With continued representations to the government by the new Canadian Hospital Council, a body more representative of Canadian hospitals, various tariff changes were made and public hospitals were saved considerable expense.

For many years the CHC continued to meet only as a council and at two-year intervals. A frequent issue was the question of meeting annually, not just in council but with an annual convention. Earlier the answer was clear: the four-thousand-mile ribbon of hospitals, the limited funds available for travel, the concentration of many delegates on provincial problems, the danger of harming the exhibit income of various provincial and regional associations and the proximity of American hospital organizations with their large and established conventions – all contributed to delay an annual and national convention.

In 1953 the council changed its name to the Canadian Hospital Association and five years later an assembly held in Toronto (convened at that time by the pressing issue of hospital insurance) marked the beginning of annual meetings.

Over the years the Canadian Hospital Council (Association) has achieved a great deal. It did much to strengthen the provincial and other associations and to collate the experience gained in all provinces. One of its lasting achievements has been the stimulus given to hospital workers across the country to get to know each other and exchange ideas. The council did more than has been generally recognized in helping the federal government lay a sound foundation for the development of hospital insurance. It has instigated or supported legislation and regulations at both federal and provincial levels and has assisted in defeating measures considered harmful.

A strong medium for the interchange of information has been developed in *The Canadian Hospital*. This monthly journal was started as a private venture in 1924 by Charles A. Edwards of Toronto. There were no hospital magazines in Canada (and only a few in the United States) and there was little contact from province to province except through supply houses. Edward's business acumen was soon rewarded, an adequate amount of advertising developed, and the journal thrived.

A crisis occurred in 1935 when a large publisher proposed to start another hospital journal. This competition would have been disastrous for the still-struggling *Canadian Hospital*. The situation was resolved when the Canadian Hospital Council made the journal its official publication. A few years later the publication was given outright to the CHC by Mr Edwards, who continued as advertising manager until his retirement in 1963.

Other publications of the Canadian Hospital Council (Association) have included the annual *Hospital Directory* and the *Canadian Hospital Accounting Manual*. The original edition of the latter volume resulted from years of work by Rev Father Verreault, Murray Ross, Percy Ward and others of the CHC and James C. Brady and others of the Dominion Bureau of Statistics. During the 1950s and early 1960s Walter Dick of Moncton, E.F. Bourassa of Regina, Earl Dick of Saskatoon and their associates on the CHA Committee of Accounting and Statistics did some excellent work in producing revised editions of the manual.

The Blackader Library was established as a memorial by Dr A.D. Blackader of Montreal to his son, Capt Gordon H. Blackader, who was killed in the first world war. In 1945 the Canadian Medical Association donated this fine collection to the Canadian Hospital Council when I left the secretariat of the CMA to work full time for the council.

In 1951 the Committee on Education was established and since then the council (and later the association) has sponsored an ambitious educational program. The extension course in hospital organization and management was followed shortly by a course for medical record librarians. In subsequent years a course in nursing unit administration (jointly sponsored by the Canadian Nurse's Association and the CHA) and other programs in hospital departmental management, hospital food service supervision and hospital administrators development have been introduced. These courses have been remarkably successful by any standard but especially so in a country whose regional hospital needs are so varied yet are met by a basically common program. Some of the courses are conducted separately in English and French, but the content is essentially similar.

As already mentioned, the council changed its name to the Canadian Hospital Association in 1953 and had, in 1958, held its first national assembly. By 1968 the time was ripe – some thought overdue – for a national convention. The executive committee, with Chaiker Abbis as president, decided to introduce a full-scale program, directed not only at the official delegates determining national policies but at the individual registrant more interested in addresses on current topics and extensive exhibits. It meant a lot more secretarial work for Dr B.L.P. Brosseau, the executive director, and his staff.

The Canadian Hospital Council (Association) has had many fine leaders over the years, all of whom have made enormous contributions not only to the work of the organization but in other positions, hospitals and regions. Its presidents and executive directors from 1931 to the time of writing are listed in Appendix C.

In fleshing out this brief history of the Canadian Hospital Council (Association), the names of several dozen men come to mind. Perhaps more than any other, the name of George Findlay Stephens stands out.

Few men in the administrative field in this country have made such a massive contribution as did George Stephens. A 'triple-threat' man when he was captain of the formidable McGill football team, he graduated in 1907 and later served with the RCAMC in England and France. After the war he was assistant to Dr A.K. Haywood at the Montreal General Hospital for six months and then was appointed superintendent of the Winnipeg General Hospital. He quickly became a dominant figure in Manitoba and the Prairies generally, was elected president of the American Hospital Association for 1932 to 1933 – the first Canadian so honored – and a fellow of the American College of Hospital Administrators in 1933. Thanks to Dr Stephens' efforts, Manitoba was the first province to have Blue Cross in the late 1930s.

In 1940, he returned to Montreal to become administrator of the Royal Victoria Hospital at a time when it was facing some real problems in reorganization and in adapting some of the earlier construction to changing needs.

It was George Stephens' lot to be president of the Canadian Hospital Council (1939 to 1945) at a time when the war effort was making it exceedingly difficult to carry on the work of the civilian hospitals. The hospitals everywhere were asking the Canadian Hospital Council to help them get priority or approval at Ottawa. As council president, George Stephens took his responsibilities seriously. Yet he was capable of lighter moments; as part of his war effort he tapped the many sugar maples on the grounds of the Royal Victoria Hospital to make maple syrup – and with calm good nature took the ribbing he got.

A tall, erect man, he wasted little time on small talk or dictation. If possible he replied on a corner of the original letter, usually with a blunt 'yes' or 'no.' If several items required a reply, he would add a succinct marginal comment such as:

'1. Yes; 2. No; 3. ?; 4. You decide.'

The strain of carrying on the work of the national council as well as of directing his own hospital's undertakings eventually took its toll. In 1945 he suffered a cerebral thrombosis from which he never fully recovered. He continued some of his duties under considerable difficulty but suffered a terminal relapse in 1947.

An oversight which still, after twenty-five years, seems unforgivable was that the government of the day did not recognize his services when the extensive list of civilian recipients of the Order of the British Empire was announced after the second world war. One or two OBE's were awarded to a wide range of national organizations. The Canadian Hospital Council was *not* on the list, despite its intensive efforts during the war years. Hospital people in all parts of Canada were upset by this lack of recognition, particularly as Dr Stephens had been permanently stricken largely because of his constant efforts to keep the civilian hospital system going with attenuated rosters of personnel and increasingly obsolete equipment. He made superhuman efforts to keep in close contact with many hospitals and attempted to help them meet their research objectives, training programs and other war requirements. Although Dr Stephens himself was too modest to mention the oversight, I went to Ottawa to discuss the matter with the Minister of National Health and Welfare. He expressed regret but stated that it was thought that recognition of the Canadian Medical Association and the Canadian Nurses' Association would adequately cover the hospital field. He stated that several other serious omissions had been brought to the cabinet's attention and that these would be contained in a supplementary list with Dr Stephens' name among the first. No such supplementary list was ever issued.

It was the American Hospital Association which recognized his wartime services when it awarded him its much-coveted Award of Merit in 1946.

In his memory the Canadian Hospital Council set up the George Findlay Stephens Award in 1949 to recognize outstanding leaders in the hospital field. This highest award of the Canadian Hospital Association is awarded 'not more frequently than once in each calendar year and not necessarily that often' for 'noteworthy service in the realm of hospital administration.' Priority is to be given to consistent service and leadership over the years rather than for a single contribution or achievement. It is to be in recognition of administrative contributions rather than for clinical or research achievement. Priority is given 'for personal efforts to advance the efficiency and welfare of Canadian hospitals, to improve administrative methods, to develop national or provincial associations, to provide assistance to other hospitals, to foster better public relations, for the furtherance of social and other legislation relating to hospital care and for efforts to advance administrative policies in general.'

Recipients of the George Findlay Stephens Memorial Award have been:

1949 A.K. Haywood, MD, British Columbia
1950 Fred Routley, MD, Ontario
1951 A.L.C. Gilday, MD, Quebec
1952 A.F. Anderson, MD, Alberta
1953 G. Harvey Agnew, MD, Ontario
1954 A.J. Swanson, Ontario

1955 Percy Ward, British Columbia
1956 Mother M. Ignatius, Nova Scotia
1957 R. Fraser Armstrong, Ontario
1958 J.H. Roy, Quebec
1959 A.C. McGugan, MD, Alberta
1960 Judge J. Milton George, Manitoba
1961 Right Rev John G. Fullerton, DP, Ontario
1962 Mother M. Berthe Dorais, Quebec
1963 J. Gilbert Turner, MD, Quebec
1964 Stanley W. Martin, Ontario
1965 Judge Nelles V. Buchanan, Alberta
1966 no award
1967 Father Hector Bertrand, Ontario
1968 John Edward Sharpe, MD, Ontario
1969 no award
1970 no award
1971 Chaiker Abbis, New Brunswick

THE CATHOLIC HOSPITAL ASSOCIATION

In 1915, Rev Father Moulinier, of St Louis, Missouri, provided much of the foresight and energy necessary to found the Catholic Hospital Association of the United States and Canada – an organization designed to meet the special needs of Catholic hospitals. Its initial membership included forty-two hospitals and twenty-three individuals. By 1923, of the 674 Catholic hospitals in North America, 500 had joined the new association and the personal membership had expanded to more than 1,000.

Regional associations or conferences sprang up in many places; the first in Canada was organized in the Maritimes in 1924. Mother Audet of Campbellton, New Brunswick and Sister (later Mother) Ignatius of Antigonish, Nova Scotia, organized many meetings for the Catholic hospitals in this part of Canada in the early years. By 1933 conferences had been organized in Quebec, the Prairies and Ontario following an appeal from Mother Allaire of Montreal to the parent organization for assistance.

The Ontario conference was organized in 1931 just before the inaugural meeting of the Canadian Hospital Council. Sister Madeleine de Jesus of Ottawa and Sister Margaret of Toronto (who attended the first CHC meeting) were the first president and secretary-treasurer respectively.

The Prairie provinces conference was formed in 1932, with the Rev

Mother Laberge of Edmonton as the first president. This conference split into three separate provincial conferences after the second world war.

The British Columbia conference was organized in 1940 and the initial hospital membership totalled nine. The Rev Mother Mary Mark of Victoria and Sister Columkille of Vancouver were the first president and secretary respectively.

The provincial or regional Catholic conferences met at the same time and place as their corresponding regional hospital association convention. The Catholic delegates would attend general sessions of the hospital association convention and then adjourn to separate sessions at which they considered matters of particular pertinence to Catholic hospitals.

During the 1930s complaints were voiced that Canadian hospitals and their special problems were viewed with ignorance or indifference by the executive of the Catholic Hospital Association based in St Louis. There was within the Catholic organization a growing rift between the Canadian and u.s. membership. An incident occurred during the second biennial meeting of the Canadian Hospital Council in Winnipeg in 1933 which illustrates the growing tension.

Father Alphonse Schwitalla, speaking as president of the Catholic Hospital Association, delivered an address which sternly rejected the idea of hospital insurance. Further, Rev Schwitalla opposed any change in capital financing which might lead to greater government financial involvement or control.

Most American hospital men then (and a great many, still) were opposed to the 'socialistic' notion of state participation in the voluntary hospitals. But many Canadians thought otherwise. After the meeting I was approached by the mother superior of a western Canadian order who indignantly informed me of her opposition to Father Schwitalla's views. She was not prepared to risk an open rift by opposing the president of her organization on the floor of the meeting. But she wanted her order's opposition noted.

Another complaint that fostered discontent was the fact that *Hospital Progress*, the journal of the Catholic Hospital Association, contained virtually no Canadian content and ignored the bilingual needs of this country.

In 1935 the Archbishop of Quebec, his Eminence J.M. Rodrigues Cardinal Villeneuve, convened a meeting of Catholic hospitals of Canada in Ottawa to discuss the situation. There was some talk of establishing two executive committees of the hospital association – one for Canada and one for the United States.

After further negotiations and some experimentation a Canadian Council of the Catholic Hospital Association was set up in 1939. Several months later the name of this new body was changed to the Canadian Advisory Board of the Catholic Hospital Association. Rev Mother Margaret of Toronto and Sister Dorais, then of St Boniface, were the first chairman and secretary respectively of this new group.

The career of Sister Dorais illustrates the fact that so many of the Sisters have displayed unusually competent executive ability. Although born in Quebec, Sister Dorais was brought up in Saskatchewan before joining the Grey Nuns in Montreal. She was the first secretary of the Catholic Hospital Association of Canada and its president on two occasions, 1943–1945 and 1961–1962. She has been president of the Catholic Hospital Conference of Manitoba; on the executive board of the Associated Hospitals of Manitoba; vice-president of the Greater Winnipeg Hospital Council; on the board of directors of the Quebec Hospital Service Association and of l'Association des Hôpitaux de la Province de Québec; and on numerous other boards and commissions. In her order she has been administrator of St Boniface Hospital; Provincial Superior, Alberta and Northern Saskatchewan; Treasurer General, Grey Nuns of Montreal; and consultant on general administration to the order. She is also a fellow of the ACHA. It is no wonder that Sister Dorais received the George Findlay Stephens Award in 1962.

My most vivid impression of Sister Dorais in action was in 1945 when Dr Heagerty's committee at Ottawa was working out the proposed hospital insurance legislation. The right of the Canadian Hospital Council to speak for all of the hospitals across Canada, as it had endeavored to do, was sharply challenged by a prominent clergyman in the educational field who insisted upon Catholic hospitals having a separate voice at federal and provincial levels. This upset the federal committee. Sister Dorais, who had helped to work out the brief of the Canadian Hospital Council, decided quickly to go with me to Ottawa. As president of the Catholic Hospital Association of Canada, she stated that in matters involving the morals of practice in Catholic hospitals or matters involving the welfare of nurses and others in their charge, the Catholic Hospital Council of Canada would speak for itself; in matters of a general nature, such as hospital insurance and legislation in general, the Canadian Hospital Council, of which they were a part, would speak for them. Her statement settled the matter.

In 1941 the Canadian Advisory Board of the Catholic Hospital Association changed its name to the Catholic Hospital Council of Canada and eventually to the Catholic Hospital Association of Canada in 1954. Until 1952, the CHAC remained closely affiliated with the Catholic Hospital Association of the United States and Canada.

Two outstanding presidents managed the affairs of the Catholic Hospital Council during the forties – first Sister Dorais, and from 1945 to 1952 Father Hector Bertrand, who worked for the council and Catholic hospitals with the energy of a multitude of men.

Father Bertrand burst upon the hospital scene in Canada immediately after the second world war. A Jesuit of formidable energy with natural abilities as a leader, he threw himself into hospital work with a vengeance. Within a few years he had made a lasting impression on hospitals in Quebec and throughout Canada as a whole with his work on the CHA. Always deeply concerned with education, Father Bertrand has been vice-president (administration) of the University of Sudbury for a number of years. He has maintained his interest in hospital affairs, however, and is currently the chairman of the committee on educational programs of the CHA. His work in the hospital field has been recognized with two recent awards. In 1967 he received the George Findlay Stephens Memorial Award of the CHA and in 1970 he was granted an honorary fellowship of the American College of Hospital Administrators.

Succeeding presidents and executive directors of the CHAC are listed in Appendix F.

The Catholic Hospital Council (Association) of Canada has had an excellent working relationship with the Canadian Hospital Council (Association) for many years but during the early forties there was a real danger that there would be a split between the two. At that time, a Quebec faction in the CHCC challenged the right of the Canadian Hospital Council to make representations on behalf of Catholic hospitals to the Federal Advisory Committee on Health Insurance. Fortunately wiser counsel prevailed and the Catholic hierarchy took a hand in the discussions. Bishop (later Cardinal) James McGuigan of Toronto saw the dangers at once and agreed that all hospitals should be united in one strong organization. As mentioned, Rev Sister Dorais was exceedingly helpful and deserves much credit for holding the two groups together.

Over the past decade or so the Catholic Hospital Association of Canada and Catholic hospitals generally have undergone an identity crisis as an increasing number of people within the Catholic Church have questioned the care of the sick by church-operated institutions. It is argued that the fundamental objective of the church should be to pass on the faith, an objective which is not being accomplished by the modern hospital.

Catholics, like persons of all faiths, demand hospital care as a right from the state and are primarily concerned with the quality of care rather than whether it is delivered in a religious institution.

In addition, membership has declined considerably in some orders during the past two decades as fewer young women have chosen the religious vocation and others have left. The average age of Sisters in some orders has increased substantially and there has been difficulty keeping some hospitals staffed.

On the other hand few would dispute the desirability of maintaining the Sisters in the hospital field at least on a personal level. Furthermore, unless the Sisters own and operate their own hospitals they will have a considerably diminished influence over medical issues in which they see crucial moral overtones – for example, abortions.

The Catholic Hospital Association of Canada has studied these and related issues and has served as a valuable forum to discuss the future role of the Catholic hospital.

THE BRITISH COLUMBIA HOSPITALS' ASSOCIATION

The British Columbia Hospitals' Association has the distinction of being the oldest existing hospital association in the country. Not surprisingly, much of the credit for its inception must go to Dr Malcolm MacEachern, its first president from 1917 to 1918. Dr Mac enthusiastically encouraged the establishment and development of hospital councils and associations, not only by helping to set a good example in his own province, but by his immeasurable contributions across the continent. Another early leader in British Columbia was Dr Horace Wrinch, the renowned surgeon of the Skeena and founder of the Wrinch Memorial Hospital in Hazelton. Dr Alf Haywood, F.F. Reid, Judge Swencisky, J. Abrahamson and Harvey Taylor are other names which come immediately to mind for their work in furthering the objectives of the BCHA. One figure stands out, however. Percy Ward was the association's secretary from 1948 to 1958, and was respectfully and affectionately known in BC as 'Mr Hospitals.'

These leaders guided the organization through a half-century of slow but continuous growth and today 105 public hospitals enjoy membership. These include all public general and some federal and provincial hospitals. Private hospitals have had their own organization since 1963.

Beginning as a trustee and administrator organization, the association has extended services to a wider range of hospital workers. The first full-time executive secretary was appointed in 1958. Kenneth Conibear served in that capacity until 1962 when he was succeeded by the present executive secretary, Duncan Bradford.

In the past decade there has been a marked increase in association activities to include much broader consultative services, particularly in regard to labor relations and regional planning. Educational programs, institutes, conferences and other counselling services have also flourished.

THE ALBERTA HOSPITAL ASSOCIATION

'In the opinion of a large number of superintendents and other hospital workers in Alberta, the time is now ripe for the organization of all hospitals and kindred institutions in the province into an association ...'

This declaration from a notice dated September 21, 1919, heralded the inaugural meeting of the Alberta Hospital Association. Convened on the campus of the University of Alberta in Edmonton in late October of that year, the meeting was organized primarily by the Very Reverend Dean J.E. Murrell Wright of Lethbridge and Dr James C. Fyshe of Edmonton. These two gentlemen were subsequently elected the association's first president and secretary-treasurer respectively. Dr Albert E. Archer of Lamont was elected vice-president at the assembly and succeeded to the presidency the following year.

A Methodist (United) Church medical missionary to the Ukrainian settlement around Lamont, north of Edmonton, Bert Archer was a born leader for the medical and hospital associations in Alberta. His clinic and the hospital at Lamont were noted for the quality of their work and they soon began to serve patients from far afield. He became president of the Canadian Medical Association and chairman of its general council. Later, as chairman of its committee of economics he did much to clarify the thinking of this organization on the controversial and emotional issue of medical health insurance and was a great help to the Canadian Hospital Council's Committee on Hospital Insurance. He had an interesting eccentricity. A constant traveller in later years, he practically never carried overshoes despite winter snow and slush. His great work at Lamont has since been carried on by his younger associate, Dr Morley Young, FRCS(C), who, like Dr Archer, has made tremendous contributions to organized medicine and to hospitals.

The objectives of the initial association included the standardization of every hospital and training school for nurses in Alberta, and the securing of increased provincial government grants and subsidies in order to obtain better facilities, especially for the aged, the tuberculous and those suffering from chronic diseases.

In November 1920 representatives of the newly established municipal hospitals considered their interests and problems sufficiently differentiated to form a separate association. At its first annual meeting in Edmonton, the Alberta Municipal Hospital Association elected James M. Taylor as its president. Serving in this capacity for some twenty-three years and later as president of the Associated Hospitals of Alberta, this greatly respected leader from Hanna made many worthwhile contributions to the alleviation of problems encountered by municipal and other hospitals.

Although the two associations continued to function separately throughout the 1920s and 1930s, some municipal hospitals were members of both; pressures to merge the two groups were often intense. As early as 1925 a resolution of the Alberta association called for amalgamation. Annual meetings were often held conjointly and I remember many gatherings which featured stimulating papers and lively discussions. The two associations usually met together and then the municipal section held its own session.

Efforts to achieve a coalescence continued and by 1943 the Associated Hospitals of Alberta had been created. James Barnes of Calgary was the first president of the new structure.

A major milestone was the establishment of the Alberta Blue Cross Plan in 1948. Built on the mode of the Edmonton Group Hospitalization Plan, Blue Cross became rapidly popular in other parts of the province. After the introduction of provincial hospitalization in 1959, Alberta Blue Cross continued to provide coverage not included in the provincial plan.

Not until 1959 did the Associated Hospitals of Alberta (which reverted to its original name, Alberta Hospital Association, in 1966) provide for the employment of full-time staff. Murray Ross, who had given such valuable service at the CHA as well as in hospitals in Saskatoon, Lamont and Edmonton, became the first full-time executive director. This and other progressive changes were brought about under the forceful leadership of Judge N.V. Buchanan, president of the Alberta association from 1952 to 1954 and again from 1957 to 1960.

Chief Judge Buchanan was a native of Manitoba but has spent most of his eminent career as a lawyer and jurist in Alberta. For many years chairman of the board at the Archer Memorial Hospital in Lamont, he contributed countless extra hours not only to that institution but also to the Alberta and Canadian Hospital Associations. Judge Buchanan worked closely with Joe Monaghan and others at Alberta Blue Cross for many years.

I cannot conclude this short history of the development of hospital associations in Alberta without mention of one of the province's great pioneers, Dr E.A. Braithwaite. Born in the Channel Islands in 1862, Braithwaite emigrated to Canada in 1884 and joined the RCMP (then known as the North West Mounted Police). He was made a hospital sergeant and treated the wounded militiamen at the battles of the Riel rebellion of 1885 in the Northwest Territories. In 1890 he took his medical degree from the University of Manitoba and practised first at St Albert, then about twenty miles from Edmonton, and later at Lac Ste Anne, northwest of Edmonton. It was at St Albert that Dr Braithwaite performed a mastoidectomy with a sharpened spike and a carpenter's mallet. In his later years he was medical inspector of hospitals for Alberta and did much to develop improved standards of care before being succeeded in 1938 by Dr Angus McGugan. He was also chief coroner for the province for eighteen years. In this connection he told of doing one of the earliest medico-legal autopsies in the province on a hillside on a body suspected of encountering foul play. The native population, disapproving of autopsies or perhaps fearful of someone discovering the truth, kept shooting at the doctor from the cover of bushland. Brathwaite Park, south of the university campus in Edmonton commemorates the life and work of this great pioneer who died in 1949.

During the past decade the programs and projects of the Alberta Hospital Association have increased dramatically. Educational seminars and institutes for every type of hospital worker have proliferated under association sponsorship. The association has become involved in all the major issues facing hospitals and hospital personnel during this period and has kept its members informed through a regular newsletter, *HospitAlta*, begun in 1962.

THE SASKATCHEWAN HOSPITAL ASSOCIATION

During the summer of 1919 a few leading members of the staff of the General Hospital in Weyburn, Saskatchewan, resolved that the time was opportune to form a provincial hospital association following the example of British Columbia a year ealier. They approached the administration of the Regina General Hospital, which in turn contacted the thirty-seven hospitals in the province to arrange an organizational meeting in Regina. This first annual meeting of the Saskatchewan association held on October 8, 1919, attracted thirty-one persons from sixteen hospitals. Although there are indications that R.H. Williams was the chairman of the first convention, records listing the first president are apparently non-existent. However Charles E. Barton of Regina, a former president of the Canadian Hospital Association, and executive director of the SHA for some years now, believes that the first president was either a Dr Mitchell or a Dr Stephens. The secretary for more than twenty-five years was George Patterson, administrator of the Regina General Hospital. Patterson, a genial and accommodating man, ran the association from his hospital office.

The available records, dating from 1930, indicate that the special problem of the day was that of the indigents. Where residency could be established the hospitals tried to collect from the municipalities but they, in turn, had no money during the depression. The association members were concerned that hospital costs were rising to about $2.50 per day. Something had to be done to control spiralling expenditures, the members felt.

The first full-time officer of the association was E.V. 'Wally' Walshaw who worked from his home in Saskatoon. Later, after Walshaw's death in 1956, the association opened an office in Regina with a secretary and stenographer.

A major change in the association took place in 1966. Earlier emphasis had been upon the presence of administrators on the board of directors, largely because of their personal 'know-how' of hospital operation. During the presidency of William Holtby of Moose Jaw the principle was reversed; the new concept provided for a trustee-oriented board with few administrators serving. A further revision of the by-laws in 1967 provided for direct representation of the regional councils.

The association has become a busy one. Trustees are taking more interest in provincial matters than ever before. Nurse and dietary consulting services are available to member hospitals, as is competent labor-management advice. An association committee has been helpful in achieving province-wide acceptance of uniform nurse salaries. Province-wide pension and group life plans have been sponsored by the association.

In association with the government, the regional councils and the administrator's association, a strong and diversified educational program has been developed. Institutes of an educational nature have been held annually, and the correspondence course in hospital administration at the University of Saskatchewan invited to participate. A study is being made towards developing a health science library service for Saskatchewan hospital personnel. Group purchasing has been undertaken by the Southwest Regional Hospital Council and the service has been extended to member hospitals of the other regional councils.

THE MANITOBA HOSPITAL ASSOCIATION[3]

The strong man in the hospital field in Manitoba during the 1920s and 1930s was Dr George F. Stephens. This greatly respected administrator of the Winnipeg General Hospital, along with Dr Gerry Williams of Winnipeg and Joe Metcalfe of Portage la Prairie helped to organize many of the early annual meetings, some of which were held in conjunction with the provincial nurses' association.

The primary topic of concern at most of the early annual meetings was hospital financing. The hospital trustees and administrators in Manitoba watched with interest the development of group hospital insurance in the United States. In the late thirties Dr Stephens, who was also active in the American Hospital Association, sought and won the support of Winnipeg community leaders in sponsoring the first province-wide Blue Cross plan in Canada. It commenced operations in January 1939 and stimulated other such plans across the country.

Although the association did not have a full-time paid officer until 1950, a degree of continuity was given by E. Gagnon of St Boniface and Walter Bell of Souris, secretary and treasurer respectively for many years during the 1930s and 1940s. Herman Crewson, present executive director of the Manitoba Hospital Association, writes:

Not only did the secretary not have an office provided, it is said that he did not have a briefcase and demonstrating his desire for the association to purchase one for him, Mr Gagnon appeared at meetings with the association's material wrapped in brown paper and tied with ordinary string or binder twine. Mr Gagnon finally got his briefcase, however.

During the late forties an increasing number of rural hospitals, established by newly created municipal districts (similar to those in Alberta and Saskatchewan) made heavy demands on the Manitoba Hospital Association consultative services. The individuals on the MHA board of directors simply could not meet all the requests within a reasonable time period and it was decided in 1950 to appoint a full-time executive director. The first person to hold the appointment was Paul D. Shannon.

In 1954, largely due to the efforts of Shannon and his successor, R.G.

---

3 Originally and currently known by this name, the association used the title Associated Hospitals of Manitoba from 1950 to 1965.

Goodman, and with the financial support of the Kellogg Foundation, the association began a report accounting program for small and rural hospitals. This service provided hospitals with data necessary for them to negotiate with the third-party paying agencies (Blue Cross and the different levels of government).

Promoting and supervising these developments during the 1940s and 1950s were such individuals as John Gardner of Dauphin, Christine McLeod of Brandon and (until 1950) Don Cox of Winnipeg. Two remarkable gentlemen, Dr Owen C. Trainor and Judge Milton George, deserve special recognition. Dr Trainor was a federal MP at the time of his death in 1956 and had been active not only with the Manitoba association but with the CHC, an organization he served as president from 1951 to 1953. Milton George was a graduate of the University of Manitoba and was a major force behind the building of the hospital at Deloraine, Manitoba, the town where he practised law. (In later years he moved to Morden where he continued his work with hospitals, serving as board chairman for many years.) He served on numerous Manitoba and national committees and, at one time or another, was chairman of most. He was co-ordinating chairman of the first meeting of the Western Canada Institute when it met in 1946; a member of the health advisory board of the province; and a commissioner serving on the hospital accreditation commission. For these and a host of other services to Canadian hospitals, Judge George was awarded the George Findlay Stephens Memorial Award of the CHA in 1960.

In the late fifties, as in other provinces, the Manitoba association was concerned primarily with the introduction of government hospital insurance. Various individuals, including Mr Goodham, left the association to work for the new Manitoba Health Services Plan. G.A. Pickering of St Boniface, then on the board of the Associated Hospitals of Manitoba, became the first commissioner of hospitalization.

During the sixties the association greatly expanded its consultative services and in 1965 introduced a computerized management information system. This program presently serves seventy hospitals in the province. The potential for long-term savings through this and other centralized services is considerable.

Another ambitious and worthwhile project in recent years has been a full-scale program to assist hospitals in attaining accreditation. This has been run with the support of the medical and nursing professions and with the financial assistance of the federal government.

Various other educational, group purchasing, and employee relations services were greatly expanded in the late 1960s.

THE WESTERN CANADA INSTITUTE

The hospital associations in the western provinces lacked sufficient resources to conduct an educational program or full-scale convention such as the larger Canadian and American associations were able to sponsor. Holding joint sessions with provincial nursing associations helped to some extent. In order to provide hospital personnel with an opportunity to hear and meet the outstanding leaders in the hospital field from North America and Great Britain, the hospital associations of British Columbia, Alberta, Saskatchewan and Manitoba formed the Western Canada Institute in 1946.

Each association took turns organizing the institute, which was held in conjunction with the annual meeting of the host association. The first was held in Winnipeg and was a great success largely due to the efforts of Judge Milton George, Don Cox and Dr Owen Trainor.

Don Cox was one the stalwarts of the western Canada hospital scene. From 1932 to 1942 he was first assistant secretary manager and then secretary manager of the Winnipeg Municipal Hospitals. He was a founder of the Western Canada Institute for Hospital Administrators and served a term as president of the Upper Midwest Hospital Conference. Later he moved to the west coast and for twenty years served the British Columbia government as deputy minister of hospital insurance until his retirement in 1972.

Trustees and administrators from the western provinces made a point of going to the institute and some years as many as 2,000 registrants participated. The pressing issues of the day were thoroughly discussed and hospital personnel were stimulated by these ambitious conferences.

By 1967 the annual conventions sponsored by the individual provincial associations had improved substantially. At that time the Canadian Hospital Association decided to sponsor a full-scale convention at its annual meetings and for these reasons the Western Canada Institute was dissolved.

However, the sponsoring body of the institute, the Western Canada Council, continued to function and in September 1968, with the financial assistance of the Kellogg Foundation, began an educational program for health care administrators. The council has been primarily concerned with co-ordinating the activities of the existing educational programs in hospital administration available in western Canada. Besides the four provincial hospital associations, membership in the council has been expanded to include the division of health service administration of the University of Alberta and the Canadian Hospital Association.

THE ONTARIO HOSPITAL ASSOCIATION

I have referred already to the short life of the original Ontario Hospital Association, the group that was organized in 1902 and apparently disbanded by 1904.

At the turn of the century Ontario hospitals were in a financial squeeze of large proportions. Government grants towards the care of indigent patients had fallen from thirty to eighteen cents per day; at the same time the actual costs of caring for patients had climbed from forty or fifty cents per day to eighty cents and occasionally as high as one dollar. Something had to be done.

A meeting was called for February 1902 in Toronto and an association was formed. The purpose of the group, according to its minutes was: 'To procure increased government aid for the maintenance of indigent patients in the public hospitals of Ontario; also to get county and civic aid as well (to further) general promotion of hospital work.' The first officers were: *President*, E.C. Gurney, Toronto; *Vice-Presidents*, Charles O'Reilly, MD, Toronto, J.O. Featherstone, Ottawa, B.W. Robertson, Kingston, Adam Bucke, London[4], George Roach, Hamilton, H. Malcolmson, Chatham; *Secretary-treasurer*, John Ferguson, MD, Toronto.

Any member of a hospital board could become a personal member of the association for one dollar. By 1904, when the second meeting was held, twenty-five hospitals had joined (the hospital membership fee was not recorded) and thirty individuals. The association's income was reported as $195 and expenses were $78.09.

We know that the original OHA met a second time, in 1904, but beyond that no further information about the organization exists. It is possible, however, to surmise that the 1902 meeting of the OHA was aimed primarily at hospital trustees. The 1907 meeting of the Canadian Hospital Association – briefly alluded to at the beginning of this chapter – was directed at superintendents.

Whatever the cross-currents of opinion were at the time is of little consequence today. Both the early organizations withered and disappeared with little written record of their existence. It is testimony to the tenacity of a good idea that both a Canadian Hospital Association and an Ontario

4 Adam Beck, later Sir Adam, of London and the father of hydro power in this country, was noted as a vice-president in 1904. Could Bucke and Beck be the same person? The records were hand-written and confusion might have resulted between the names of Beck and Dr R.M. Bucke, a noted psychiatrist, also from London.

association – spiritual descendants of these early, aborted groups – continue in vigorous existence today.

The present Ontario Hospital Association was formed at a meeting of an invited group of hospital trustees and superintendents in December 1923. They met at the Toronto Academy of Medicine, then on Queen's Park Crescent at Grosvenor Street, on the suggestion of Dr Fred W. Routley, then Ontario director of the Canadian Red Cross.

At this meeting it was agreed to organize and to hold a first convention in February 1924. Lieutenant-Colonel William Gartshore of London was elected president; Mrs H.M. Bowman of Women's College Hospital, first vice-president; Dr Edward Ryan of Rockwood Hospital (Mental), Kingston, second vice-president; and Dr Fred W. Routley, secretary-treasurer. By the time of the 1924 meeting membership in the new organization was thirty-nine hospitals and individuals. One hundred and six people registered at the convention. By November 1928, all but 15 of Ontario's 147 public hospitals had become members. By the end of 1970 all of the public general, convalescent and extended care hospitals were members, as well as most of the provincial mental hospitals. The registration at the annual convention in 1970 had risen to 7,996.

The Ontario association has had a commendable history of achievement. It has always been strongly supported by hospital trustees and this has been a considerable factor in the respect with which the association has been regarded at Queen's Park. Its quest for better hospital legislation has been noticeably successful.

At its annual meetings the program is broken down into detailed specialties and interest has been maintained across a broad spectrum of hospital personnel – trustees, accounting and bookkeeping personnel, pharmacists, medical record librarians, engineering staff, dietetic workers, hospital auxiliaries, medical technologists, occupational therapists, physical therapists, radiological technicians, social workers, tuberculosis workers, purchasing department staffs, housekeeping and laundry personnel and many more. Tickets to the annual banquet, the highlight of the convention, are so much in demand that they are issued on a quota basis to member hospitals.

Perhaps the association's most notable achievement was the early development and operation of a Blue Cross plan in 1941.

In 1947 the association purchased the old United Church Training School on St Clair Avenue West in Toronto. Within a short period of time even this large building proved insufficient to house the 700 persons employed to administer the plan, for by the early fifties the plan, under the direction of David Ogilvie and assistant director and comptroller, C.A. Sage, was serving the needs of 2,250,000 Ontario subscribers.

In the late 1950s a new high-rise headquarters building was conceived by a committee under the chairmanship of Mrs Charles McLean, a former OHA president and chairman of the board of the Toronto Women's College Hospital. The building was planned to be large enough to handle the staff required for the obviously forthcoming provincial plan of hospital insurance. Provision for housing provincial employees was made because at one stage in the negotiations Premier Leslie Frost told the committee that, for the first few years at least, the government would like the plan to be administered by the OHA and its Blue Cross plan. Later, the government reconsidered and decided to operate its own plan.

By this time the plans for the new building were well advanced. A happy solution was reached when the province agreed to take over the Yonge St property, continue with the same architects and complete the building for the use of the Ontario Hospital Services Commission. With this episode settled, the association then went on to build a new home in Don Mills, a suburb to the northeast of Toronto. This building was officially opened in 1961, but OHA activities expanded so much in the next decade that the association has again moved, this time to a new fourteen-storey building nearby.

Besides offering a wealth of educational conferences, institutes and extension courses, the OHA has offered a statistical and consultant service and recently has co-operated with the Ontario College of Physicians and Surgeons to conduct surveys and make recommendations for small rural hospitals. As in other provinces hospital-government relations have become more intense and the association has been kept busy representing the hospitals.

This extra workload has been very capably supervised by the Ontario Hospital Association's executive directors.

No history of the OHA – even a truncated version such as this – can be written without mention of the work of Arthur J. Swanson.

Arthur Swanson was born in Moose Jaw and served with distinction in the first world war. In 1930 he was promoted to administrator of Toronto Western Hospital. He was possessed of formidable energy and it was in large part his doing that Toronto Western Hospital assumed its present place as a leading scientific institution. No matter how tight the money supply, if his medical staff wanted better equipment, Swanson somehow found the money. He was tough but always fair; his medical staff loved him for it. His personnel were loyal beyond belief. Without really trying – it was just part of his personality – he developed a rapport with every staff member that would be the envy of a labor-management consultant.

One day as he and I were rushing out to a luncheon appointment for which we were already late we passed a group of employees pitching horseshoes on the lawn. One man threw a ringer as we passed. Mr Swanson paused and then threw out the challenge, 'Bet you two bits I can beat you.' I held the fifty-cent bet while Swanson and the employee pitched a few ends. Amid great hilarity, Swanson lost and I paid off the wager. Whether Swanson lost on purpose I cannot say. I *do* know that his few minutes and twenty-five cents did a great deal to win him friends.

He became a member of the OHA early in his career and served as its president from 1937 to 1938. In 1951, when Dr Fred Routley died, Arthur Swanson was wooed away from his beloved Western to become executive secretary of the OHA. It was his drive that brought Blue Cross to Ontario at an early date. When the Ontario Government set up the Ontario Hospital Services Commission, Swanson was chosen by Premier Leslie Frost to be its first chairman. It was a formidable task and one which required every bit of administrative skill that could be mustered. It is a tribute to his ability and to those whom he recruited to help him that the provincial plan was rapidly accepted by the hospitals.

Another 'mover-and-doer' of Blue Cross in Ontario was R. Fraser Armstrong, a civil engineer from New Brunswick, who was for many years superintendent of the Kingston General Hospital. For many years he was a director of the Ontario Hospital Association, and served a term as its president. A founder of the Canadian Hospital Council, he became its president in 1949–51, served on many committees, and became a fellow and regent of the American College of Hospital Administrators. He received the George Findlay Stephens Memorial Award in 1957.

The OHA was – in a very real sense – 'born' at the first annual convention of 1924. But not many of the delegates who attended realized how close the birthday came to being a day of tragedy.

The program committee had arranged for me to demonstrate a simplified technique for whole blood transfusion which involved a piece of equipment which had been developed by one of my clinical chiefs in New York. A donor had been selected and the necessary blood grouping had been done by the hospital laboratory and checked by the assistant pathologist in charge. The gallery and the floor of the operating room were filling rapidly. An acknowledged 'fusspot' regarding detail, I decided to occupy the last minutes before going in by doing another check, a direct crossmatch. To my horror, the clumps of reddish, agglutinated cells were distinctly visible without the use of a microscope.

The bloods were absolutely incompatible. The young lady donor would have received the first syringeful all right. But by the time the turnscrew would have been turned and a second syringe of blood partly withdrawn, she would have given a gasp and been beyond help.

(I was never able to find out to my own satisfaction why the laboratory had passed the blood for compatability. The director of the laboratory was absent at the time. But techniques for blood matching were not fully mastered, and there was conflict of terminology between the then-used Moss and Jansky classifications. There were no A, B, and O groupings then.)

The committee was by this time asking if we were ready to go in. My knees were knocking so badly that I needed time to think. My intern, Dr John Fawcett, saved the day. As a 'universal donor,' he volunteered for the demonstration. (We had more faith in the safety of using a so-called universal donor or of being a universal recipient then than we had later as more research revealed subgroupings and other causes of reaction. We *did* believe then that one might get a reaction from a universal donor but the blood would not cause death.) Dr Fawcett got on the table, I went on with my descriptive discourse, the transfusion went fine and the delegates never realized what a tragic situation they could have witnessed.

HOSPITAL ASSOCIATIONS IN QUEBEC

The Montreal Hospital Council, founded in 1926, was for some years the only hospital association in Quebec. The sessions of the council were bilingual and superbly organized and a number of administrators in other parts of the province requested permission to attend. Their hospitals were considered associate members. These, I recall, included Jeffrey Hale's Hospital of Quebec City, Sherbrooke Hospital and Barrie Memorial at Ormstown.

Over the years the council has achieved a great deal in co-ordinating practices, internal regulations, charges, and so on, and in developing a good camaraderie among the executive personnel. The prominent figures in the early days included Dr A.K. Haywood of the Montreal General, Dr L.A. Lessard of Notre Dame Hospital, Montreal, W.R. Chenoweth of Royal Victoria, Dr A.L.C. Gilday of Montreal General (western division) and J.H. Roy of l'Hôpital St Luc. Roy was president of the council from 1937 to 1958.

Responding to the needs of the large numbers of Catholic, French-speaking hospitals in Quebec, the Catholic Hospital Association of the United States and Canada assisted in establishing a conference of the CHA in Montreal in June 1932. Rev Sister (later Mother) Allaire of Montreal, Rev Father (later Monseigneur) Victorin Germain of Quebec and Rev Father Ivan d'Orsonnens of Montreal did a great deal of work in helping to set up the conference and organizing its annual meetings. This group was originally known as the Conference of Quebec Hospitals, but a differentiation was necessary when a second conference based in Quebec City was formed in 1935.

The work of the conference was shared among many Sisters over the years and one hesitates to mention some and not others. However, Mother Allaire of Montreal and later Mother Ste Jeanne de Chantal of Quebec were exceptionally active in conference affairs.

As already mentioned, in 1947 a Jesuit priest, Father Hector Bertrand, established le Comité des Hôpitaux de la Province de Québec. With the blessing of the Catholic hierarchy and his own remarkable talents, Father Bertrand organized numerous programs and projects which did much to raise the quality of patient care in many hospitals. The committee started out as a joint committee of the conferences of Montreal and Quebec and was primarily concerned with organizing and conducting the annual Congrès des Hôpitaux Catholiques de la Province de Québec. Before long, however, the committee came to represent all but a few Catholic hospitals in Quebec, all Catholic hospitals in New Brunswick and many in Ontario. The agenda and exhibits of the congress were unsurpassed in Canada and registration rose during the 1950s to more than five thousand.

In 1948, Father Bertrand initiated an ambitious educational program for French-speaking hospital workers. Organized as a series of workshops each lasting from one to six weeks, the courses provided excellent instruction. Where French-language instructors were not available, leading experts from across Canada and the United States were imported. Many lectures, essays, textbooks and other important documents were translated into French.

In 1955, Father Bertrand founded *L'Hôpital d'aujourd'hui*, a monthly French-language hospital journal. *Canadian Hospital* had periodically published articles in French, but this was inadequate to maintain the interest of French-speaking hospital personnel, much less keep them informed. *L'Hôpital d'aujourd'hui* fulfilled those functions and has continued to thrive. After Father Bertrand left in 1963, Roland Levert, associate director of the committee's hospital administration course, became editor until the end of 1965, when Jean-Claude Deschênes assumed control. As the activities of the committee were being transferred or phased out in the early 1960s, l'Association des Administrateurs d'Hôpitaux de la Province de Québec provided assistance and assumed control of the journal.

One of Father Bertrand's fervent desires was to see the majority, if not all, of the hospitals in Quebec obtain accreditation. He has done more to raise and achieve hospital standards in Quebec than any other person.

In 1958, largely at the instigation of the Montreal Hospital Council, an effort was made to form an association whose membership would include all hospitals in the province. The Quebec Hospital Association was set up, not to replace completely the individual hospital groups, which were to continue to attend to matters affecting their respective interests, but to deal with issues and problems affecting all hospitals – especially hospital insurance and other financial concerns. Marcel Piché and Dr Gerald LaSalle were the first president and executive director respectively. Dr J. Gilbert Turner, A.H. Westbury, Dr Paul Bourgeois and Eugene F. Bourassa were a few of the leading figures in the early years.

The Quebec Hopital Association grew rapidly for a few years. Then its membership levelled off at about seventy hospitals – just less than half of all hospitals in the province – by 1962. Most Catholic hospitals retained membership in the Catholic conferences and le Comité des Hôpitaux. Some joined the QHA or maintained dual membership, but by and large the two groups remained distinct.

In the meantime the Quebec government had decided to inaugurate a hospital insurance program under the Hospital Insurance and Diagnostic Services Act. Naturally, officials of the provincial department of health sought the advice and recommendations of the hospitals collectively and urged them to make a joint submission. In 1960, le Conseil Provisoire des Hôpitaux Catholiques, soon to be re-named la Commission Générale des Hôpitaux Catholiques, was created by the Catholic conferences to work out a joint presentation with the Quebec Hospital Association. Over the next two years the two bodies co-operated on a variety of presentations to the government, especially those respecting budget proposals. In 1962 the Catholic Hospital Association of Quebec was formed to replace la Commission Générale and encompass the activities of le Comité des Hôpitaux. The first president of this association was Mother Maillé of Montreal. Among those who deserve credit, not only for their assistance in supporting the new organization but for past efforts on behalf of their associations, are Sister Germaine Michand of Montreal, Sister Ste-Marie-Madeleine of Montmagny, Mother Marie de Grâces of Giffard, Sister Marie Aimée de Jésus of Montreal and many others.

The Catholic Hospital Association of Quebec worked closely with the QHA on such matters as the writing of rules and regulations under the 1963 Hospital Act, a province-wide pension plan for hospital personnel and budget forms. A permanent joint committee on professional relations was established.

There was a great desire, as well as need, to amalgamate the two associations and after lengthy negotiations they joined forces in 1965 under the name of l'Association des Hôpitaux de la Province de Québec. Dr Gaston Rodrigue, previously active in le Comité des Hôpitaux, was the first president.

At present the AHPQ has some two hundred hospital members with more than fifty thousand beds. Since 1965 Quebec hospitals have faced considerable problems in labor relations and hospital budgeting and have made good use of the excellent consulting and other services of their association.

HOSPITAL ASSOCIATIONS IN THE ATLANTIC PROVINCES

Influenced by the growth and services of the Maritime conference of the Catholic Hospital Association and of hospital associations in other provinces, the progressive hospital leaders of New Brunswick, Prince Edward Island and Nova Scotia resolved to form their own association in the late twenties. In my capacity as secretary of the Department of Hospital Service of the CMA, I was invited to assist in organizing the Maritime hospitals in the spring of 1929.

Originally it was hoped that the hospitals of all three provinces would unite to form one association. However, at the last moment several key trustees from New Brunswick changed their minds and decided to form a separate association. They believed that the problems and interests of New Brunswick hospitals were sufficiently different to warrant this step. 'It was a surprise to many that the [New Brunswick] Association decided to remain a Provincial organization rather than become a Maritime one, incorporated with Nova Scotia and Prince Edward Island.'[5]

The other delegates meeting at Truro, disappointed by this decision, proceeded to form the Hospital Association of Nova Scotia and Prince Edward Island. At the first annual conference Major W.A. Fillmore of Amherst was elected president. Also on the executive was Sister (later Rev Mother) Ignatius of Antigonish, a born leader, who was the keynote

5 Extract from the first annual report of the New Brunswick Hospital Association, 1930

speaker of many annual meetings. When I think back to the early years of the CHA and the Maritime organizations, the memory of Mother Ignatius' hard work, constructive enthusiasm and endless goodwill remains fresh. She was always in the forefront of progressive hospital developments; St Joseph's Hospital in Glace Bay, Nova Scotia, of which she was the administrator for many years, was one of the first hospitals in the country to win accreditation. For several years she served on the CHA's board of directors and in 1956 was awarded the association's George Findlay Stephens Memorial Award.

Other members of that first meeting at Truro included Lauchie Currie and Herb Wright. In a part of Canada blessed with good orators (at least, that was true in the hospital associations) these two men stood out.

The Honorable Lauchlin Currie – as he was later to become – was a delegate to the conference from Cape Breton Island. He went on to become a member of the Nova Scotia legislature and eventually the minister of mines, attorney-general, minister of public welfare and minister of health. At one period, he held three of these portfolios simultaneously. Later he was appointed to be a justice in the provincial supreme court.

Herbert G. Wright was a Newfoundlander by birth but a Nova Scotian by adoption. He was a minister of the United Church of Canada and, true to the traditions of the cloth, could be counted on to support whatever was obviously in the public interest. In addition to his hospital work, Herb Wright proved his humanity by sticking by the poverty-stricken miners of Inverness in Cape Breton. He was an early president of the Hospital Association of Nova Scotia and Prince Edward Island and served on the executive of the Canadian Hospital Council as well. He was an ardent fisherman, and when the problems of his poverty-ridden parish became discouraging, Herb found relaxation in donning a pair of waders and surf-casting for striped bass. But the problem of educating his family finally forced him to leave Inverness and take other work, a second career that was cut short by his early death.

At that first Maritime meeting I can also recall the fiery oratory of the hard-hitting newspaper editor from Windsor, Nova Scotia, Jean Fielding.

The separate association formed in New Brunswick elected F.A. Reid and Colonel T.G. Loggie (both of Fredericton) as president and secretary. J. Chapman, chairman of the Moncton General Hospital and his superintendent, Miss A.J. McMaster, Sister Audet of Campbellton and Dr Hugh Farris of the sanatorium at Saint John were especially zealous in their efforts to promote the interests of hospitals in New Brunswick.

Issues discussed at the annual meetings were markedly similar for both associations throughout the thirties. 'Maritime union' was the recurrent theme and by 1937 an agreement was reached whereby the two associations were to meet conjointly every second year. In 1941, at the second joint meeting, Dr George Stephens, then Canadian Hospital Council president, and I supported the unionists; following the report of Mother Ignatius' committee recommending a unified association, the Maritime Hospital Association was formed in July 1942. Dr Joe MacMillan of Prince Edward Island, a veritable dynamo who added a great deal of color to the meetings, was elected first president of the Maritime association. Ruth Wilson of Moncton became secretary and did an outstanding job, not only in that capacity but as administrator of the Blue Cross plan in the Maritimes.

That Blue Cross organization, known as the Maritime Hospital Service Association, was formed in 1942 and 1943 under the sponsorship of the Maritime Hospital Association. The plan was administered and promoted so well that in just four years there were more than two hundred and fifty thousand subscribers. In 1948, the MHSA became one of the few Blue Cross plans in North America to operate medical and surgical insurance programs as riders to the basic hospital coverage.

The Maritime Hospital Association prospered throughout the forties and by the mid-fifties there were more than one hundred member hospitals. This included all the public general and special hospitals in the three provinces.

The advent of provincial prepaid hospital insurance in the late 1950s was largely responsible for the fragmentation of the Maritime Hospital Association, this time into separate units for each province. It was the belief of most of the hospital leaders in the Atlantic provinces that more and more issues and problems faced by the association – especially those dealing with the new insurance regulations – were of a provincial nature and could be dealt with best by separate associations. By 1962 dissolution had been largely accomplished. Although the Atlantic provinces continued to meet annually under the auspices of the Maritime Hospital Association for educational purposes, all other functions, including direct representation at the Canadian Hospital Association, had been taken over by the provincial organizations.

Newfoundland, whose citizens had become eligible for coverage by the MHSA in 1949, had not formed a hospital association prior to that date. This was due in part to the lack of resources and transportation facilities and in part, also, to the fact that the province and the Grenfell association owned most of the hospitals in the province. Many hospital staff believed that the exchange of information and ideas among hospitals via their parent organization was adequate. In addition, the staffs of the provincially owned hospitals were obviously not in a position to form political pressure groups.

By the mid-1950s some Newfoundland hospitals were sending delegates to Maritime Association annual conferences and a Newfoundland section was created. In 1962, the Newfoundland Hospital Association was formed and the first annual conference was held in the spring of 1963. Dr A.W. Taylor and Sister Mary Fabian were the first president and secretary.

In recent years the NHA has conducted an active educational program and assisted in promoting greater hospital autonomy through semi-global budgeting control of non-government hospitals. Until 1969, R.D. Moore served as executive director of the association but left in that year to join the St John's General Hospital which was transferred from government to voluntary board control.

One of the most difficult problems faced by any association in the Maritime provinces in the last decade was countering the recommendations contained in the report of the Byrne Commission. This report, commissioned by the New Brunswick government in 1963, recommended that the government assume control of voluntary hospitals. The NBHA appointed a committee under the chairmanship of Chaiker Abbis of Chatham to prepare a brief countering the report. Abbis' committee pointed out the various deleterious effects of direct government ownership of hospitals (as opposed to provincial budgetary controls). The committee also recommended that qualifications for employees in the hospital division of the Department of Health be raised to afford greater budgetary controls. As a result of this brief the New Brunswick hospitals continue to be administered by locally appointed boards of trustees.

Since dissolving the authority of the Maritime Hospital Association, the New Brunswick, Nova Scotia and Newfoundland associations have set up their own executive offices. The Prince Edward Island Hospital Association, with only nine members has, not surprisingly, decided that the appointment of a full-time executive director would be impractical.

In 1966 the old Maritime Hospital Association was renamed the Atlantic Provinces Hospital Association and continued to function as a loose federation of the four provincial organizations.[6] Although not yet as ambitious, its educational programs are in some ways analogous to those of the old Western Canada Hospital Institute.

6 The Newfoundland Hospital Association withdrew from the Atlantic Provinces Hospital Association in 1971.

NORTHWEST TERRITORIES HOSPITAL ASSOCIATION

The most recent hospital association to be formed is that of the hospitals in the Northwest Territories. In 1965, the Reverend K.A. Gaetz and Peter Verhesen were elected the first president and secretary-treasurer respectively. With only four or five member hospitals and considerable problems of transportation and communication, the programs and activities of this association have been relatively limited to this time. However, as the population of the region expands, and as the difficulties of transportation in the north ease, this association too will increase its activities.

LOCAL HOSPITAL COUNCILS

That local groups of hospitals should get together to discuss their mutual problems is but to be expected. In some instances they have been essentially administrators' conferences, dealing mainly with the day-to-day problems faced by all. Others have brought together representatives at the trustee level with greater emphasis upon capital financing, government and community relations. The term 'council' would be more correctly applied to these local groups.

The local hospital council was, in one sense, a forerunner of the regional hospital planning council which, in recent years, has developed as a means of co-ordinating programs and avoiding duplication of services. They differed, however, in that the hospital council was essentially a council of hospital representatives, usually of a city; the regional planning council has usually contained a substantial number of individuals not connected with any of the hospitals but representative of the public as a whole. It has usually been concerned with hospitals from a larger geographical area.

The first local council was the Montreal Hospital Council, but this rapidly developed into a small association as there was no provincial hospital organization in Quebec in the twenties and for some years to come. In 1958

The formation of the Quebec Hospital Association meant that the Council passed over to the Association the responsibility for all matters affecting hospitals as a whole in the province, such as membership in the Canadian Hospital Association, liaison with professional bodies and paramedical groups, holding of institutes, submissions to the Provincial Government and its agencies, et cetera.[7]

7 From the 1958 annual report of the Montreal Hospital Council.

The Montreal council continues to function as an administrators' conference, dealing with problems affecting its membership exclusively.

Two other local hospital councils formed in the thirties continue to survive. The Edmonton Hospitals' Advisory Council was a natural outgrowth of the Edmonton Group Hospitalization Plan begun in 1933. All four general hospitals participated – Misericordia, Edmonton General, University Hospital and the Royal Alexandra. Later in 1958 it was decided to unite the Edmonton and Calgary hospitals in a joint Edmonton and Calgary Hospitals' Advisory Board. This arrangement continued until 1966 when the council was dissolved. The Edmonton group then re-formed as the Edmonton General Hospitals Division of the Alberta Hospital Association.

Throughout 1935 many hospital executives, doctors and others in Toronto were actively considering the formation of a city-wide plan for group hospitalization in co-operation with the Civil Service Association of Ontario. This consideration led to the formation of the Toronto Hospital Council in January of 1936. Membership included the majority of Toronto hospitals and although the plans of the Civil Service Association did not materialize, it was proposed that the council could serve as an organization through which co-ordinated action could be taken respecting municipal or provincial legislation. The council was also seen as a group through which co-operative developments such as central purchasing, city-wide planning and a central collection system for various accounts would be possible. These ambitious objectives were never fully realized but in recent years the council – now the Hospital Council of Metropolitan Toronto – has accumulated a number of progressive achievements, most notably the development of centralized laundry and purchasing services.

Numerous other local and regional hospital councils have existed from time to time, including various subdivisions of provincial hospital associations. They have fulfilled the traditional functions of the local council and recently have begun sponsoring some centralized services.

ASSOCIATIONS OF TEACHING HOSPITALS

For many years after hospital associations were founded in all parts of Canada, it was recognized that one segment of the hospital community was not adequately served by the existing organizations: the teaching hospitals had unique problems and few adequate forums in which to discuss them. By 1958 the American Association of Medical Colleges had formed a hospital administration section and member deans could select administrators to attend the meetings. Several of the Canadian member deans took their principal administrator to that meeting of the AAMC but the administrators did not feel that the program fully met their needs.

In 1959, a meeting in Toronto of the principal administrators involved set up the Executives of Teaching Hospitals Club, a small organization which met regularly each year and is still meeting.

In the meantime the Association of Canadian Medical Colleges had established a permanent secretariat and about 1962 set up an administrators' section and administrators were invited to participate. Some differences of opinion continue as to whether the administrators should be part of the ACMC or be separate. The final decision – in 1966 – was to form a separate body, the Association of Canadian Teaching Hospitals, with authority to determine its own membership. However the ACTH works closely with the ACMC and they continue to hold joint sessions and to share a secretariat. The first chairman was Dr Arnold Swanson, then executive director of Victoria Hospital, London, and the secretary was Dr L.O. Bradley, then executive director of the Winnipeg General Hospital. Earl Dick, executive director of the University Hospital in Saskatoon, was secretary in 1970. At the time of writing there were forty-nine member hospitals.

L.O. Bradley, the ACTH's first secretary, is exuberant, witty and a tireless worker with an exceptionally wide and varied background to draw upon in his present position as executive director of the Canadian Council on Hospital Accreditation. Shortly after graduation from the University of Alberta medical school, Dr Bradley entered the medical corps of the RCAF. After the second world war he became interested in problems of hospital administration and subsequently attended the course in hospital administration at the University of Chicago. Shortly thereafter I was fortunate to obtain his services on the staff of the newly formed course in hospital administration at the University of Toronto. In 1950 he became secretary of the Canadian Hospital Council. After serving as administrator of the Calgary General Hospital from 1952 to 1956, he moved eastward to direct the Winnipeg General for eleven years. Before joining the CCHA as executive director in 1969, Dr Bradley was president of the Minneapolis Medical Center for two years.

To say that Brad has perpetually worked a twenty-hour day maintaining multitudinous other interests in hospital associations and voluntary agencies would be only a slight exaggeration. Chairman of the Canadian Medical Association Committee on Approval of Hospitals for training of Junior Interns, president of the Winnipeg Rotary Club, president of the Association Hospitals of Manitoba, chairman of the Canadian Hospital Association Committee on Education and Research, a trustee of the American Hospital Association, chairman of the Canadian Red Cross Committee on Outposts are only a few of his past titles. He was also elected first president of the Canadian Council of Health Service Executives in 1970.

A major impetus to the establishment of the Association of Canadian Teaching Hospitals was the federal government's passage, in July 1966, of the Health Resources Fund Act, a piece of legislation which set aside $500 million for the building or renovating of medical training facilities. At first, the amount of money available seemed overwhelmingly generous. But, when the pencils were sharpened and accurate calculations made, it was found that the medical schools, teaching hospitals and nurses' schools could have spent the sum easily in one year alone, let alone spread it out from 1966 to 1980 as the act stipulated. The committee appointed to apportion the funds was composed largely of representatives of the medical schools. It was only natural that the teaching hospitals should band together into an association to provide a single voice to represent their interests.

In the past few years local organizations of teaching hospitals have been formed. In December 1970, a University Teaching Hospitals Association was formed in Toronto with ten hospitals and the University of Toronto as members. An earlier proposal for a university-teaching hospitals centre with binding membership commitments was abandoned. The association is a voluntary organization, with equal representation from the hospitals which will endeavour to integrate and co-ordinate programs to maintain excellence and to eliminate unnecessary duplication. At the same time, the association respects the corporate integrity of each constituent member. The initial executive director is Claus A. Wirsig.

The Montreal Joint Hospital Institute, whose membership includes McGill University and its four teaching hospitals – Montreal General, Montreal Children's, Royal Victoria and Montreal Neurological – was formed in January 1971. The scope of this organization's activities has yet to be determined.

There is also an Ontario Council of Administrators of Teaching Hospitals of which Donald M. MacIntyre, executive director of the Kingston General Hospital, was president in 1970.

None of these local bodies are members of the ACTH but they are represented through their member hospitals which ensures close relationship.

INTERNATIONAL ASSOCIATIONS

Canadian hospitals have always been heavily influenced by the activities of the American Hospital Association; as already mentioned, the original association was known as the Hospital Association of the United States and Canada and a number of Canadian hospitals were and still are members of the AHA.

For a long time the AHA conventions have been the most extensive and well organized of any hospital associations. While many of the sessions have had little relevance for Canadian hospitals, others have been very helpful and informative. The American Hospital Association has met four times in Canada – in Toronto in 1908, 1931 and 1939 and in Montreal in 1920. The 1931 meeting was held in conjunction with the inaugural meeting of the Canadian Hospital Council. The 1939 meeting was to have been held at the same time as a congress of the International Hospital Association but the outbreak of the second world war prevented the joint meeting.

This latter organization was founded in the late twenties. Through the efforts of Dr E.H.L. Corwin, Dr S.S. Goldwater, both from the United States, Dr Réné Sand of Belgium, Professor J. Tandler of Austria and many other international figures in the hospital field, an international hospital congress was held in Atlantic City, New Jersey, in 1929. This meeting proved so successful that a second congress was organized two years later, at which time it was decided to form a permanent International Hospital Association. This organization continued to meet every two years until 1939. Its post-war successor was the International Hospital Federation which continues at the time of writing.

Although both of these bodies have had only a limited impact on Canadian hospitals, the meetings have broadened the perspective of those in attendance and assisted hospital men to re-examine many basic assumptions. Many delegates have been government representatives, as most hospitals in a great many countries are owned and directed by the government. Their outlook on various problems has been different from that of spokesmen from the United States, Canada and Great Britain where the hospital systems have been largely voluntary. (In Great Britain the state took over in 1948 at which time the British Hospital Association ceased to exist.)

Although the international organization has never met in Canada, as previously noted this country was scheduled to host a congress of the International Hospital Association in 1939.[8] Previous to this time there had been a growing disillusionment with the attempts of German delegates – with Nazi affiliations of which they openly boasted – to direct the affairs of the association. The association was looking to America for financial support

8 The International Hospital Federation did finally meet in Montreal in June 1973.

but the Nazi group insisted upon dictating the programs and general policies. At the 1937 meeting in Paris, the annoyance with the German delegates in the secretariat led to a confrontation.

At the final session of the conference the dam burst. The English-speaking delegates had been the guests that day of the American Hospital in Paris and generous care had been taken that they should become well acquainted with France's finest liquid nourishment. It was an excellent conditioner for the afternoon's exercises. The president, Dr Réné Sand, noted Belgian public health authority, author and master of five languages, tried valiantly to calm the emotions but to little avail. '*Je suis désolé*,' he kept repeating. A delegate from the Irish Republic, bouncing beside me summed it up: 'To my Irish heart, this is just like home.' The Germans were voted down and greater powers were given to the host country.

It was because of this rift that the CHC, with AHA assistance, wanted to put on an unusually good program and heal the distrust and animosity rapidly descending over the western world. But our plans came to naught when war broke out.

The International Hospital Federation was formed in 1947 largely due to the efforts of Dr Sand and Captain J.E. Stone of Great Britain. During the 1950s it had to struggle along on a meagre budget. Gradually member-ship increased and brought in more funds for the IHF. A full-time staff was appointed and *World Hospitals* began publication in the early 1960s. Study tours have been inaugurated and along with the biennial convention have become more ambitious and better organized.

4
Hospital personnel
The evolution of responsibilities

It has often been stated that the most important determinant of quality of care in any hospital is the extent and quality of training received by the personnel who work there. This applies particularly to doctors and nurses but is also true for paramedical, administrative and non-medical personnel. As various pressures – new discoveries in medicine, rising costs, new administrative techniques, shortages of personnel, unionization and a growing public demand for more and better health services – as these pressures have altered the responsibilities and interrelationships of the providers of hospital care, so they have affected the content and standards of the training of hospital workers. While conditions of employment in the hospital have been continually changing over these past fifty years, so too, the standards of education and training have been constantly rising.

PHYSICIANS

Central to the delivery of health care within the hospital and without is the physician. Although the hospital has traditionally been regarded as the 'doctors' workshop,' it has become increasingly the workshop also of nurses, pharmacists, and dozens of other paramedicals. The physician remains the predominating medical expert in the hospital but it is only with the support and assistance of the entire health team that he can hope to deliver superior health care.

While depending to an ever-increasing extent on paramedical workers, the physician has become increasingly specialized in his field of medical expertise, thus raising further problems in co-ordinating and integrating medical services.

Both these developments are directly related to the remarkable advances in medical science and knowledge, advances which have also had profound repercussions for the education of doctors. The freshly graduated MD has become 'the generalist's generalist' and further specialization is imperative even for family practice. Graduation is only the first step in a doctor's training; attendance at continuing education programs, conferences, symposia and the like has become a physician's lifelong obligation if he is to keep abreast of medical developments. Unlike the nineteenth century 'diploma mills' south of the border, Canadian medical schools were – with only minor and short-lived exceptions – affiliated with or attached to universities from their inception. Furthermore, the distinction between granting a degree and licensing to practise was always strictly maintained in Canada; at no time did medical schools have licensing powers, powers which have always been reserved for provincially created licensing bodies.

For many years each province set its own standards and doctors licensed to practise in one province were ineligible elsewhere. Following the persistent efforts of Dr Thomas Roddick, the Medical Council of Canada was established in 1912 to facilitate reciprocity of medical licensure among all provinces and to help improve standards of medical education across the country. Although this body has never possessed any legal licensing authority, it has conducted annual examinations, success in which has been required by most provincial bodies.

Large hospitals treating a great variety of illnesses, especially among those unable to afford private doctors, were well-established as classrooms for the teaching of the clinical sciences by 1920. In fact, the Montreal Medical Institution, the first medical school in Canada, (shortly to become the Faculty of Medicine at McGill University), was established in 1823 by the four physicians of the Montreal General Hospital. These pioneer doctors gave their students a great deal of practical experience in the hospital.

By 1920, the time was ripe for the teaching of medicine to come to flower in Canada. In 1910 the Flexner report on medical education in North America had been highly critical. Johns Hopkins Medical School had set a high standard that other universities were striving to emulate; the Rockefeller Foundation was bestowing grants with generosity. These factors in combination prompted the University of Toronto to appoint, in 1920, the first full-time professor of medicine in Canada, Dr Duncan Graham. (In fact, Professor Graham was the first full-time medical professor in what was then known as the British Empire.) Other full-time appointments followed shortly at Toronto and at McGill.

There has always been resistance by some doctors to full-time (that is with minimal or no private practice) appointments to the medical schools; the argument has been that full-time professors would lose touch with the 'practical side of medicine.' For this reason, and in order to employ the best experts available in each specialty, a great deal of medical teaching has been done on a part-time basis by appointing to the active staff of teaching hospitals leading physicians in the community. Certain senior appointments to the active staff of teaching hospitals affiliated with a medical school have been the traditional prerogative of joint hospital-university relations committees in order to ensure some measure of control for the medical school over the clinical teaching of its students.

Although the medical student has been introduced to the clinical sciences after the second year of medical school, at least until recent years, the majority of such students have not obtained significant clinical experience until their internship. This position is of such obvious importance that the Canadian Medical Association had set up standards for the approval of internships; but the prevailing practice in the twenties and thirties was for graduating students to apply to as many of the approved hospitals as possible, hoping to land one position out of many. A prudent administrator or intern committee might fill a quota, only to find that some (or occasionally all) of the students accepted had decided to work in some other hospital. Some non-teaching hospitals lost out badly.

In 1938 the Canadian Association of Medical Students and Interns (CAMSI) was formed with Dr P.F. McGoey as its first president. Although created to deal with a variety of issues of concern to students and interns, the most pressing problem of the day was to bring some order out of chaos in the appointment of interns. To improve the situation with regard to the graduate internships (as opposed to university controlled, final-year internships), CAMSI, with the assistance of the Canadian Medical Association Department of Hospital Service, evolved a matching arrangement. Graduating students listed in order the hospitals they desired. The hospitals listed in order the students they desired. The two lists were matched and students assigned. The arrangement worked out remarkably well. To carry out the program CAMSI requested that there be set up a Canadian Intern Board of three members, one member each from the Canadian Hospital Council, the CMA Department of Hospital Service and CAMSI.

CAMSI promoted student interest in other areas, through presentations to the CMA with which it became affiliated in 1946, sponsorship of educational conferences, and publication of the CAMSI *Journal*. In 1970, the organization was dissolved and the intern placement program taken over by the Association of Canadian Medical Colleges.

This latter body was established in 1943 with the express purpose of securing a supply of medical officers for the armed services while at the same time maintaining and improving the quality of medical school teaching. Since the second world war the ACMC has conducted research into a wide range of problems facing medical education such as the supply of qualified teachers and the costs of medical education in schools and teaching hospitals. Through its membership in the Association of American Medical Colleges, the ACMC participates in the accreditation of medical schools in Canada.[1]

The teaching hospitals which participate in the education of medical students, interns and residents have had to cope with a special problem. Should emphasis be on patient care and welfare, as in the case of non-teaching hospitals, or should the primary emphasis be upon teaching and research? In many instances the question is largely academic. But when it does arise, as it does constantly, it is bothersome in such matters as the selection of patients, the length of stay of certain patients, the cost of running the hospital, the privacy of patients, the privileges of non-teaching doctors and the number of beds available to them, and many others. In cities where alternative hospitals for non-teaching doctors are limited, the allocation of beds has caused much concern. The increasing number of geographic full-time staff doctors in many teaching hospitals has become part of the whole problem. Also the tremendous increase in residents in teaching hospitals, now receiving salaries far beyond what was paid a few years ago, can only be met by the hospitals if the government insurance program provides the finances.

University representation on the boards of teaching hospitals has been the traditional means by which the medical school promoted its educational objectives in such hospitals.

In some instances the health sciences centre has developed as:

a comprehensive health educational complex incorporating a university-owned hospital as the basic clinical teaching facility. This has many advantages from the University point of view, most prominent being its ability to place teaching

1 Accreditation of Canadian and U.S. medical schools is undertaken by a joint committee of the American Association of Medical Colleges and the American Medical Association.

priorities ahead of patient care priorities. It is a self-limiting advantage, however, because few hospitals (and medical staffs) have a captive market of sufficient size and diversity. In large centres especially, hospitals must compete for admissions from the community and for referrals from other practitioners. At the same time, the health sciences centre hospital can never be so large that it will adequately provide clinical material in all the specialties and sub-specialties of medicine. The medical school must have affiliation arrangements with other teaching hospitals for graduate training even if not for the undergraduate programs ...[2]

The University of Alberta Hospital in Edmonton has served as the main teaching hospital of the university since the early twenties. Others, such as the University Hospital in Saskatoon (dating from the mid-1950s) and centres still under construction in Vancouver, Hamilton and London are more recent. The Centre Hôspitalier de l'Université Laval in Quebec City and Sunnybrook in Toronto were both transferred to university control from the Department of Veterans Affairs in recent years.

Another recent means by which the conflicting objectives of the university and its teaching hospitals have been reconciled is the association of teaching hospitals and the medical school, through which lines of communication are established on a continuing basis. This has helped to promote a much higher degree of understanding, co-operation and co-ordination among all participants.

People often seem to fall into two categories: those who take a dim view of any major change in the status quo, and those who avidly support almost any idea or proposal as long as it is new. In between there is a broad grey area (in which you, the reader, and I, the author, naturally belong); people there are all for new ideas yet at the same time are careful to keep their feet on the ground. The result is like an ever-turbulent sea; humanity is always restless, going with the wind of the day, yet providing an underlying strength and basic steadfastness which, if properly directed and controlled, can be used to much advantage.

In hospital-medical relationships over the years there has been turbulence and many a storm but the hospitals and the profession continue to function together more efficiently than ever in the past. This association has existed for centuries and will go on for centuries more. It is one which must be flexible, able to change with the times, weather storms and always provide an efficient service to those who need it. Where personal interests

2 Claus A. Wirsig, 'Bridging Hospital-Medical Relationships,' *Newsletter No. 11*, International Hospital Federation Teaching Hospital Committee, July 1971

are at stake, be they financial or those of status; where the welfare of society is concerned; where large amounts of public funds are involved and where scientific procedures and socio-economic factors are constantly changing; in these circumstances there are bound to be frequent changes of relationship, some misinterpretation and a real necessity to put emphasis upon the long-range trends and the public interest.

Over this past half century the relationship has been, on the whole, a satisfactory one, most of the occasions for differences of opinion having been in recent years. The major areas of contention have been admitting privileges, the payment of radiologists and other physicians working almost exclusively within the hospital, and medical staff representation on the board.

In most communities, particularly smaller ones, practically all doctors have some hospital connection, either on the active or the courtesy staff. In smaller centres, a doctor who practised in a nearby village likely would be appointed to the courtesy staff. In larger centres with medical schools the practice has varied. Many teaching hospitals have fairly large courtesy staffs with the doctors' privileges limited to private and semi-private accommodation. A few have allowed non-teaching courtesy staff to have limited public (now standard) ward privileges. Some have non-teaching as well as medical school appointees on the active staff. Some have allocated a certain percentage of beds to the teaching group; others have required all public ward beds to be available for teaching even though the patient be under another doctor's care. In most of the smaller and medium-sized hospitals in the between-the-wars period, any active staff member had full privileges, including surgery, if he wished to exercise them.

The teaching hospitals in Montreal tended to be closed, with the active and associate staffs sometimes supplemented by a limited number of well-qualified doctors with courtesy privileges. Other doctors were affiliated with non-teaching public or private hospitals. In the early 1960s my associates and I made an extensive study of the hospital facilities in Metropolitan Toronto; the various regional medical societies told us that practically all of their members had some hospital connections.

The relationship between hospitals and staff doctors has not always been smooth. A number of factors has contributed to the friction.

The earliest influence was that of the standardization (accreditation) program which did not limit privileges *per se*, but which did require better pre-operative study, more complete records, regular staff meeting attendance and the frank discussion of deaths in hospital. These requirements resulted in more efficient staff work and the withdrawal of operating room privileges from some staff members.

Another factor affecting the relationship was the certification of specialists by the Royal College of Physicians and Surgeons of Canada. While the overall effect of certification was to improve the quality of care, particularly in surgery, it did cause, for one generation at least, considerable resentment on the part of many older practitioners. They had done much of their own surgery for years and then found themselves deprived of these privileges by new staff regulations in their local hospital. The Royal College had not instigated these staff restrictions but, with an accepted definition of who is a specialist, this definition became the basis on which an individual was granted major privileges in the hospitals.

The next development naturally followed. Major hospital privileges were gradually restricted to a relatively small number of doctors, not only in the larger hospitals, but in many of seventy-five to one hundred beds, and in some that were even smaller. For the doctors not so privileged, it was the easy way out to vent their resentment on the hospital, its trustees and administration. This was hardly fair, for the regulations were proposed almost invariably by the medical staff and merely ratified by the trustees. It was alarming to note in my many contacts across the country how critical the 'average' doctor was of the hospitals because of his limitation of privileges and for the increased amount of paperwork which had to be done on the patients he did care for in hospital. This resentment was frequently voiced at medical association meetings and, for a period, even produced a 'town vs gown' situation in association elections.

The general practitioners were most affected by these changes. Many, and particularly those who had fled the medical limitations in Great Britain, foresaw the general practitioner being squeezed entirely out of all but rural hospitals. Fewer medical students were planning to go into general practice.

In quite a number of hospitals of large or medium size there developed 'general practitioner' sections which gave the family physician a rightful status in the general hospital, usually with the elected representative or head of the service sitting on the medical advisory committee. A section of the medical by-laws and regulations defined the extent to which major procedures could be undertaken by the members of the section. In some cases the privileges of each member were defined; when he completed some special course – in anaesthesiology, for example – his privileges could be extended accordingly. The committee members in charge of the service – family physicians – have usually been so anxious to make the arrangement work that they have tended to bear down harder on their colleagues than would have been likely had the supervision been by a specialist.

In keeping with this recognition of the place of the general practitioner in the urban hospital was the movement to set up a national body. In 1947 the Canadian Medical Association named a committee under Dr Wallace Wilson of Vancouver to consider the feasibility of setting up an organization to elaborate and encourage the improvement of standards for the general practitioner. Generally there was strong support for incorporating this body as a section of the Canadian Medical Association. However, it was decided finally that the objectives of the proposed organization would be served best if it were independent.

In March 1954 the College of General Practice was founded, with Dr Murray Stalker of Ormstown, Quebec, as president and Dr Victor Johnson, a former rural general practitioner from Lucknow, Ontario, as executive director. Much of the rapid growth during the early years was due to Dr Johnson's energetic leadership. Membership requirements have gradually become more stringent and at the time of writing included a requirement of a minimum of one hundred hours of approved postgraduate study in each two-year period – a most commendable feature. The college has pressed for more intensive undergraduate training in family practice, as it has become increasingly obvious that the newly graduated doctor is no more qualified to practise general medicine than many of the traditional 'specialties.' To more correctly reflect the emphasis placed upon family practice, the name of the organization was changed in 1969 to the College of Family Practice. The college, from its early years, has been served by a very readable and well-edited journal, *The Canadian Family Physician*.

During the 1930s and the early 1940s, there was a diversity of opinion respecting the financial relationship between radiologists and the hospitals. Like surgery, radiology was associated in the public's mind with mystery, magic and miracles. The average person credited the X-ray machine with visionary powers never claimed for it by Roentgen or his successors. (I can still recall the awe with which I viewed the moving bones of my hand and arm when I was taken as a child to see the first X-ray machine installed in Toronto.) In addition, the radiology department was usually the hospital's only division operating at a profit. Naturally the division of that profit became a contentious matter. Various plans for splitting it were put forward but none worked to the entire satisfaction of either party.

At the same time as the radiologists and the hospitals were arguing out their differences, the staff pathologists, psychiatrists and anaesthetists were demanding similar concessions. The hospitals, sorely pressed for funds in the days before provincial hospital insurance, found their share of the profit most useful and actually necessary to operate the extensive public wards and the out-patient department, maintained at much below cost. Hospitals were accused of practising medicine. They denied this and pointed out that radiologists' incomes were getting out of line. The patient came to the hospital department, not primarily to the radiologist, and the radiologist, unlike most of the clinical men, enjoyed a monopoly – and so continued the argument. As radiological work on non-admitted patients increased the volume of work – and the profit – radiologists in larger centres set up operation in medical office buildings and urged the profession to channel the outside paying clientele to these private offices, which many did. Another financial arrangement was urged, and began to be adopted, whereby the hospital agreed to provide space, equipment and maintenance for a part of the charges and the radiologist took the rest. Sometimes the radiologist, taking a bigger share, supplied the equipment and the technical staff. The three main radiological associations on the continent and the American Hospital Association worked out a basis of agreement which looked good on paper but which could not solve some of the problems at the local level. As a member of that committee, I sat through some frank discussions. The mutually agreeable conclusions later had their recognition resounded by the specialty societies.

The pathologists were in somewhat the same position and asked for a comparable arrangement. Pathologists' incomes were still quite low at that period before insurance plans met the charges; the free work often outnumbered the paying items, which in turn were kept minimal because of the cost. Their case was not quite comparable, however, because although the pathologist had to supervise and bear the responsibility, a great number of the laboratory tests were done by technologists. The psychiatrists and anaesthetists also insisted upon being independent contractors and wanted their contracts revised.

Many problems were involved. What is the practice of medicine? Can the profession insist upon setting a fee in a hospital-based department regardless of the rights of the hospital? Has the government the right to step in and adjudicate the apportionment of revenue? Could the department be made available to any qualified radiologist acceptable to the hospital, as is the operating room? Should the radiologist or other specialist working entirely in the hospital with hospital facilities submit his fee apart from the charges of the hospital?

These questions were debated endlessly but they lost their impact in Canada when provincial hospital insurance came into force. The new budget arrangements for hospital operation established overall requirements; hospitals no longer had to fight for every penny to meet their losses on low-income services.

The question, however, is still a very live one in the United States. In 1959, the American Hospital Association prepared a 'Statement on Hospital and Physician Relationships in Anesthesiology, Pathology, Physical Medicine, and Radiology' for the guidance of its member hospitals in both countries. In 1965 the American College of Radiology issued a statement of policy reaffirming, among other points, that the professional fee must be separated from the hospital's charges.

By the thirties more and more Canadian hospitals were including representatives of the medical staff on their governing boards. Of course, practising doctors had been board members for years but most of them did not sit as representatives of the staff. In some cases they were appointed by the local municipal council and in other cases represented a donor's estate. The board of Nicholl's Hospital in Peterborough, Ontario (later to become the Peterborough Civic Hospital) was composed of representatives from each Protestant church in the community, a stipulation of the donor. It seemed very appropriate to the various congregations to choose a doctor from their membership to sit on the hospital's board. I have never sat down with a board so heavily weighted with medical men. And a clear-thinking board it was, with such men as Dr Stewart Cameron, who was a leading figure in the preparation of the first comprehensive study of nursing in Canada, the Weir Report of 1932.

Not all hospitals were as fortunate as Nicholl's Hospital. Frequently the advice of medical members of the board was criticized by other staff members. One chairman said to me that his board had decided to disregard all medical opinions relating to board actions and depend on their own 'horse sense.' This was unfortunate for many decisions do require the special knowledge of a medical person. Some have made excellent and conscientious chairmen, as, for instance, the late Dr Norman Bragg of the Brantford General Hospital.

With the better staff organization stimulated by the standardization program of the American College of Surgeons, more hospitals were developing medical advisory committees made up of the heads of the medical services. Many hospitals were arranging for the chairman of the committee to be a member of the board, sometimes on a non-voting basis.

A long step forward was made in Ontario when the then deputy minister of health, Dr B.T. McGhie, included in the regulations pertaining to the Hospital Act that an official representative (the president or chairman) of the medical staff be named to the board. This action met with considerable opposition in some areas, for the appointees were invariably busy men. The late Dr D.E. Robertson, chief surgeon of the Toronto Hospital for Sick Children, was a case in point. Dr Robertson was nationally known for his fine surgical work and was international news for almost two weeks in the mid-1930s when he and two companions were entombed in an abandoned mine in Moose River, Nova Scotia. Dr Robertson phoned one day and let me have it as follows:

' Say, Harvey, I understand you were behind Barney McGhie in foisting this silly regulation on us,' he said. 'I'm out almost every night now on some committee or other and this is the last straw. I am not the slightest bit interested in getting mixed up in others.'

We discussed the importance of having doctors understand more fully the problems confronting the board of trustees and I made this suggestion:

'Eddie, will you note today's date and phone me a year from today and tell me how you feel about it?'

'I certainly shall,' he said, 'and I'll have wasted a lot of time in the meantime.'

Time passed and I forgot the incident. One day Dr Robertson was on the phone.

'You asked me to phone you.'

'No, Eddie, there must be some mistake. I put in no call for you.'

'Oh yes you did,' he replied, 'exactly one year ago.'

Then I recalled my request. His comment was a surprise.

'I want to tell you this has been one of the most rewarding experiences I have ever had. I had no idea of the extent of the board's problems and I took real pleasure in helping solve them.'

Dr Robertson went on record as favoring the arrangement, emphasizing its particular value to the medical staff itself.

Many in the hospital field have recommended that no member of the medical staff of the hospital be eligible for election or appointment to the board of governors except as representatives of the medical staff. This would certainly save the official medical staff opinion being beclouded by contrary private medical opinions. Others have not favored this restriction on the ground that it would deny the board the assistance of some most helpful board members. As with so many issues one could see reason in both viewpoints, but, from long observation in many situations, the reasons for the restriction seem to outweigh the disadvantages.

DENTISTS

Traditionally dentists have treated most of their patients in their private offices. However, there have been situations where dentists, and especially dental specialists, have relied on the hospital for facilities to perform highly complex and difficult procedures.

Dentists have been valuable members of hospital staffs and their position is now generally recognized and assured to a much greater extent than in the 1920s and 1930s. At that time their status was not acknowledged in some hospitals even though they devoted much unremunerated time to clinic service. Their ministrations were appreciated but as they were not licensed medical practitioners, they could not be on the staff and were not invited to staff meetings in such hospitals.

In some hospitals, even though a dentist was on the active staff – sometimes even as chief of dental department – he was not called in for the resetting and wiring together of a fractured jaw. Although the fragments usually reunited readily, the patient often could not chew food and had to go to a dental surgeon for extensive dental work. This usually involved otherwise unnecessary extractions and dependence upon dentures.

The dental profession was much concerned over this situation, taking the viewpoint that the interests of the patient warranted a joint participation of the medical surgeon and the dental surgeon, the latter to ensure that proper occlusion or 'bite' would be preserved. The workmen's compensation boards came also to be much concerned with the expensive dental follow-up and, where possible, insisted upon early dental consultation. Fortunately, in the vast majority of hospitals this problem has been eliminated.

These situations regarding dentists prevailed in hospitals across the continent. As a result the American Hospital Association in the 1930s set up a committee under my chairmanship to study the relationship of dentists to hospitals. The recommendations of this committee did much to rectify the situation and clarify the role of the dentist within the hospital.

There are no reliable statistics on how many hospitals have organized dental departments or out-patient services. In 1970, however, the Canadian Dental Association listed twenty-nine hospital dental departments which had instituted the high standards of the CDA accreditation program or were in the process of doing so. In all of these hospitals the chief of the dental department sat on the medical advisory committee of the hospital.

A growing realization of the possibilities of medical complications arising from a variety of dental procedures, especially those involving general anaesthesia, has resulted in increasing numbers of patients being treated in hospital clinics. Another factor which occasionally has strained the dental resources in hospitals has been the unfortunate provision in provincial hospital insurance plans for coverage of certain dental work only if it is done in hospitals as opposed to a private office. Regulations which encourage patients to seek more elaborate dental work in more expensive facilities than are necessary must be eliminated. Perhaps the ultimate solution lies in universal dental insurance, although one suspects that relative shortages of dentists and dental hygienists will make this impractical for some time to come.

N U R S E S

Nursing has always been a basic requirement of hospital service and much of the progress made in hospitals during this half-century has been in terms of improved nursing care. It is not my intention to record the history of nursing over these past fifty years – this story has already been told. Rather I shall attempt to outline some of the trends and developments in nursing as these have paralleled advances in medical science and affected hospital administration.

Nursing service has always been inextricably tied with nursing education – the product of the educational system determines the quality of the nursing service. It is interesting to note how the pendulum has swung from emphasis on service through apprenticeship to an emphasis on education with clinical experience. A fact which is sometimes overlooked is that the philosophy of nursing education has come full circle: the original emphasis of the Florence Nightingale School was on education through ward practice.

In colonial days, the French hospitals in settlements along the lower St Lawrence River had inherited the nursing traditions of the long-established hospitals in France. They were never well-endowed financially but were reduced to a poverty level after France withdrew from Canada. The hospitals in the English communities were suffering from the nursing decadence which had followed the action of Henry VIII in taking over the hospitals in England. This was part of the sad situation which faced the thousands of immigrants who came to Canada during the 1800s suffering from cholera, typhus, tuberculosis, smallpox and other illnesses.

The rise of modern nursing, paralleling the development of modern medicine, began with Florence Nightingale. Her influence following the Crimean war spread when the Nightingale School of Nursing at St Thomas'

Hospital was founded in 1860 in London, England. This school was established primarily for educational purposes and applicants were accepted as students.

In 1873, schools of nursing built upon the Nightingale system were established in North America. The first was at the Bellevue Hospital, New York, followed in 1874 by the first in Canada, the Theophilas Mack School at the General and Marine Hospital in St Catharines, Ontario. These were followed in 1881 by the Toronto General Hospital School of Nursing and the Winnipeg General Hospital School of Nursing, both in 1887. Largely philanthropic in purpose, these schools did not differentiate clearly between the objective of supplying a good nursing service for the hospital and that of developing a good educational system in the school. In many cases these aims were considered identical.

It soon became an almost universally accepted principle that a school of nursing was indispensable in operating a hospital, and although hospitals set up schools emulating what they believed was the Nightingale system, one important factor was missing. The Nightingale School had been originally organized as an independent institution, self-supporting and separate from the hospital. Unlike the original school, the control of these developing schools was with the hospital, the apprenticeship system flourished and the educational needs of the students were frequently subordinated to the service needs of the hospital. Poor co-ordination of classroom and bedside teaching, long hours and much night duty (often without proper supervision) not only lowered the quality of the students' training but also the quality of the service they were able to give. Undoubtedly some of the earlier schools should never have existed. The experience was altogether too limited and the teaching by the medical staff and the instructor-supervisors was haphazard and poorly planned.

It is remarkable to note that the major portion of the early graduates from Canadian schools were absorbed into private duty nursing, at first in homes and later in hospitals. As late as 1930, sixty percent of graduate nurses were employed in private duty and few hospitals employed them. Hospital nursing was done largely by students, if there was a school, or by unqualified nurses. Most training schools operated a registry of available graduates and central registries still operate in some Canadian cities.

In Canada, the qualifications and standards of training of nurses had risen substantially by 1920. Much credit for this improvement is due to the organized nursing profession. The first provincial organization to secure nursing legislation was that of Nova Scotia in 1910, although it permitted only voluntary registration and non-graduates could register. Three years later in Manitoba, better legislation was obtained which defined standards of admission to training schools, school curricula standards, conditions of registration and disciplinary powers and procedures. By 1922 all of the then nine provinces had some form of nursing registration act. Newfoundland passed its first legislation concerning nursing in 1931 and a more stringent registration act was passed in 1954.

The Canadian Society of Superintendents of Training Schools for Nurses was set up in 1907 and the following year, at a meeting in Ottawa, the Provisional Society of the Canadian National Association of Trained Nurses was established. Mary Agnes Sniveley of the Toronto General Hospital and Flora Madeleine Shaw of the Montreal General Hospital were the first president and honorary secretary-treasurer. This body became the Canadian Nurses Association in 1924.

Following the first world war, hospitals began to expand rapidly and the shortage of hospital nurses became acute. Nursing school applicants were in short supply, except in those schools which maintained the highest educational standards. Various studies and surveys were made, the most important being the Weir Report published in 1932.

This study was sponsored by the Canadian Nurses Association and the Committee on Nursing of the Canadian Medical Association of which Dr G. Stewart Cameron was chairman. Dr George M. Weir, dean of the Faculty of Education at the University of British Columbia, and shortly thereafter the provincial secretary in the Liberal cabinet of Premier Duff Patullo, directed the survey. In a letter to me in March 1932, Professor Weir said: 'The Survey was a very arduous undertaking ... Under the circumstances (eighteen months to deadline) I was obliged to work night and day at high pressure. One such experience is enough.'

It is interesting, after forty years have elapsed, to look back on some of the report's suggestions. Some indicate an early and imaginative appreciation of on-coming social change. Most seem obvious and far from radical now, although it has not been until recent years that many of the major recommendations have been implemented. To illustrate, the Weir Report recommended:

- Every training school should have at least one full-time instructor and she should act as clinician on the wards.
- Small training schools should be closed. Hospitals with training schools should have at least seventy-five beds and an average occupancy of fifty.
- An eight-hour day for nurses should replace the twelve-hour day.

- Nursing interneships should be introduced gradually.
- The training school should have a separate budget.
- The cost of nursing education should be borne by the state.
- Nurses should have a system of superannuation for their later years.
- All who nurse for hire should be subject to compulsory registration and many provincial registration acts were badly in need of amendment.

Professor Weir wanted nursing education included as part of the educational system of the province and financed on the same principle as the teacher-training schools. He was an early advocate of the specialized training of general superintendents of hospitals and recommended that superintendents of nurses have more training in hospital administration. While he defended necessary and rational discipline, he took a dim view of the overly rigid disciplinarians in some schools.

In the 1920s and 1930s nursing service was seldom adequate in hospitals, particularly on private floors and for the seriously ill patient. Dr Weir referred repeatedly to private-duty nursing as being a major objective of nursing students. He recommended that hospitals should ordinarily assume at least 50 percent more responsibility for the entire nursing care of the patient than was then generally the case.

I have elaborated many of the recommendations of the Weir Report because it was of considerable importance in its effect on the development of hospital nursing in Canada. It was studied in depth by nurses and other hospital people. Most of its recommendations were approved by the majority of nurses but profound change in any profession is usually slow in coming. In the case of nursing the apprenticeship system had become entrenched and the establishment of a pattern for change was difficult.

With this focus of attention on the educational needs of students, the consequence—reduced service to the hospital—became a concern of the superintendents of hospitals. If the hospital was to staff the wards with graduate nurses, how was the hospital to finance it, especially when balancing the budget was difficult as it was? Medical staff members were also apprehensive and even fearful; some were heard to say, 'We will have second-class doctors instead of first-class nurses.' Some nurses asked, 'Who will nurse the patient?' for they could foresee the day of shortened hours of student service. Some nurses still believed that the system of training 'how' without explaining 'why' was the only way to become a nurse.

Analysis of the content of hospital school nursing programs indicated that there were wide variations in curriculum content with little attention given to the expanding role of the services needed for practice. Nurses

were being asked to assume greater clinical and professional responsibilities as well as to perform technical services. However, ancillary staff
began to be added to take over some of the domestic duties previously performed by the student nurses. It might be noted, though, that although
many of these duties were purely housekeeping in nature, these ancillary
staff members were paid out of the nursing budget. The 'cheap hospital
labor' given by the nursing students was beginning to be looked at critically
in the early 1930s. To be sure, it was a form of indirect payment, which
the nurse gave for her education, but it was also a factor which was driving
many capable young women away from nursing, convinced that their talents and skills would be substantially wasted in housekeeping. Florence
Nightingale had made her views clear in her *Notes on Nursing*:

Nurses should not be expected, as a general thing, to do scrubbing and scouring;
it was a waste of power and poor economy to use trained people in this way ... a
nurse should do nothing but nurse – if you want a charwoman, have one, nursing
is a specialty.

In my many visits to hospitals in those early days, I frequently noticed student nurses scrubbing floors, or painting old iron bedsteads, or often functioning as messengers or porters.

Few persons had checked the balance sheet of education versus service.
The cost of nursing education was taken for granted to be offset by the services given by the student. There was little factual information as to the
true cost of nursing education and little research had been done to determine it. Beginning about 1940 various studies were undertaken in the
United States and Canada into the real costs of nursing education. These
often highlighted the extent to which nursing practice was related to nursing theory. Some of the studies showed that student nurses were being
'used' as much as 70 percent of the time for hospital service. The reports
added that nurses often performed their clinical duties without adequate
preparation.

The greater emphasis on patient care and the increasing responsibilities
assigned to nurses required more careful selection of students, as well as
changes in the educational content of the nursing courses. However, there
was a great shortage of qualified teachers and a noticeable lack of trained
supervisors. These shortages had been noted in the Weir Report but there
were few advanced courses for nurses to better prepare themselves. Bursaries, scholarships and fellowships to enable nurses to take postgraduate
work were scarce. In fact, supervisory practices were looked upon (as I

overheard more than once) as 'snoopervisory,' rather than for nurse qualification improvement or patient protection.

Beginning in 1919 university education became available for nurses
within Canada when the University of British Columbia established a five-
year course (three years of which were spent at the university). By 1926
eight Canadian universities were offering either a basic baccalaureate program or a diploma course in public health. However, the universities had
no control over most of the clinical experience of their baccalaureate students, all of whom had to attend a hospital school of nursing during their
program.

In 1933 the Rockefeller Foundation gave substantial financial support to
the University of Toronto (where a course in public health nursing had
existed since 1920) to establish an independent undergraduate school of
nursing, under the direction of E. Kathleen Russell. Within three years all
aspects of this course were under complete control of the university and
integration of theory and practice was achieved.

The other immediate and tangible consequence of the Weir Report was
the formulation and publication in 1936 of *A Proposed Curriculum for
Schools of Nursing* by a special committee of the Canadian Nurses
Association chaired by Marion Lindeburgh, director of the School for
Graduate Nurses at McGill University. This proposed curriculum set out
a logical educational program with concurrent practical experience. It was
a real endeavor to put nurse education on a par with other forms of
specialized education. With a revision in 1940, it pointed the way to a short-
ening of the three-year course as well as a revision of practical content. It
recommended that students' services in patient care should be greatly
diminished, that bedside nursing practice should be carefully examined and
that many duties redistributed to other personnel.

The implementation of many of these new policies was delayed somewhat by the second world war, as some 4,000 Canadian registered nurses
were in active service. This resulted in a severe shortage of hospital nurses
within Canada and as a stop-gap measure the training and employment of
nursing assistants became widespread. Following the war many hospital
nurses went into other branches of nursing with better employment conditions or left nursing altogether. The shortage of registered nurses persisted
and the continued and increasing employment of nursing assistants became
necessary. In 1946 the Canadian Nurses Association estimated the shortage of nurses in hospitals to be 7,000. It became obvious as never before
that in order to attract and retain the quality of nurse desired for hospital

service, more competitive salaries and working conditions would have to be offered.

The eight-hour day, less rigid residence requirements for graduate nurses, more clinical and less housekeeping duties, better salaries and more reasonable workloads were slowly introduced during the forties and fifties.

During the post-second world war era, as more and more career opportunities for women have become available, nursing has had to compete at an accelerating rate for the available qualified high school graduates. Furthermore, many nurses have been attracted to the United States where salaries have been anywhere from 20 to 50 percent higher than in Canada.

Concurrent with developing trends in nursing education was a growing debate on the future role and responsibilities of the nurse. In 1948, in *Nursing for the Future*, Esther Lucile Brown advocated two types of nurses – the professional university-educated nurse and the practical nurse. Emphasis was placed on the professional nurse but the training and the use of the practical nurse was suggested with two objectives: (1) to phase out the mediocre and undesirable schools and (2) to ensure an adequate supply of personnel to give bedside care under supervision. Dr Brown stated that the professional nurse should be trained to give good bedside care, but in addition her curriculum content should be designed largely for one of the many specialties that have since opened for nurses. One can readily see that this left a gap between the professional nurse and the practical nurse. On the one hand the practical nurse was to be limited in performance, on the other hand the numbers of university-educated nurses could not meet the demand for service.

Throughout the fifties, Dr Brown's recommendations were thoroughly debated. The future of those nurses without university preparation, but with many years of experience, who held senior administrative or teaching positions came into question. Furthermore one had to consider the important problem of mobility within the profession. University entrance requirements were generally higher than those for the diploma hospital courses and certainly higher than those for the Registered Nursing Assistants' or Nurses Aides' courses.

The 1950s in Canada were marked by numerous studies in various provinces, most of them related to nursing education and the development of two streams of nurses, one prepared in the university baccalaureate program and the other in a hospital or independent diploma program. It was becoming increasingly evident that the hospital nursing service so long relied upon and given by students under the guise of nursing education would become the full responsibility of graduate and auxiliary personnel organized under a nursing service administrator in co-operation with and supported by the hospital administrator.

Faced with a serious shortage of nurses and inspired by a belief that many of the service duties of ward care should be removed from the student nurse's responsibility, the Canadian Nurses Association, with financial help from the Canadian Red Cross Society, established in 1946 a demonstration school of nursing. The school was independent of hospital control and its students not obliged to provide hospital service. This new course, based at the Metropolitan Hospital in Windsor, Ontario, was under the direction of Nettie Fidler, previously a member of the nursing faculty of the University of Toronto. The experiment was to determine if, given freedom in theory and practice, a good bedside nurse could be produced in less than the traditional three-year period. An evaluation[3] after six years demonstrated not only that the graduates of this twenty-six month course were as competent as graduates of other nursing schools, but also that the costs per student per year were almost 25 percent lower than in other schools.

Shortly after this experiment began the Toronto Western Hospital, with a subsidy from the Atkinson Foundation, set up the first 'two-plus-one' nursing course. Classroom instruction was concentrated in the first two years and was followed by a one-year salaried interneship, featuring practical experience. The Atkinson School was watched with interest, for although closely associated with the hospital it had its own advisory council and its own budget. Under the direction of Dr Gladys Sharpe, the school had complete control of the curriculum and the students' practical experience. As with the basic university courses, students had an eight-hour day and the planned clinical content of their course was practised under supervision in the hospital situation. Although the students did make a contribution to the nursing service of the hospital, their clinical experience was assigned to complement their classroom instruction and the students were not relied upon to provide nursing service except during the third year. As with the integrated university school of nursing course, much of what had been formerly taught in the classroom was now being taught at the patients' bedside.

The success of the Atkinson School at Toronto Western Hospital

3 A.R. Lord, *Report on the Metropolitan School of Nursing*, Windsor, Ontario, 1952

meant, in effect, that the hospital had to hire other personnel to provide the services formerly supplied by the student nurses. This was hardly an overnight phenomenon, however; by 1950 many large Canadian hospitals, even those with attached nursing schools, were employing practical nurses, nursing assistants, nurses' aides and auxiliary personnel to augment the nursing staff. Also, while Toronto Western Hospital subsidized the student nurses' education to the amount of about $400 per year, this was recovered in part during the student's interne year when she performed a full day's work on the ward at a salary equal to only 70 percent of a registered nurse.

Since that time, the majority of nursing schools have become more independent of hospital nursing services, whether the school is based at the hospital, the university, the technical school or community college. Some of the smaller schools have been closed as the trend toward regional schools has increased. This trend has been most noticeable in the last decade. Regional schools have much in their favour; they are essentially educational institutions, often part of an existing college, yet they are usually also closely linked to general and other affiliated hospitals. They tap the clinical resources of many smaller and sometimes specialized hospitals, thus broadening the student's experience. Often the larger regional school can provide better instructors and facilities than would be possible in smaller schools.

For some years the future of the hospital-based diploma course has been a matter of much discussion in hospital and nursing circles. The financial considerations of former days are no longer a factor. By no stretch of the imagination could a modern training school for nurses now be termed a direct financial asset to a hospital. On the contrary, with increased educational standards and tremendously reduced clinical experience, the school is a distinct financial liability. As it happens with universal government-controlled hospital insurance, this financial factor is no longer so sensitive an issue.

The Canadian Nurses Association has stated unequivocally that the training of nurses should be controlled by educational institutions rather than service units. The Canadian Hospital Association, on the other hand, has taken the viewpoint that a well-planned and well-directed hospital-based program of nursing education has distinct advantages. What the CHA has opposed in recent years has been the efforts by many nursing leaders to have undergraduate nursing education put entirely under colleges and technical schools with hospitals being used only as areas for the practice of nursing skills. Nursing education would then be placed on the same level as any other technical course with academic work divided between the classroom and the laboratory – in this case the hospital.

In some ways, the hospitals' viewpoint is comparable to that of the medical profession with respect to health insurance. The Canadian Hospital Association's objections to the nursing association's stand has been in large part compounded of a fear of the unknown and a real concern that in completely revising the system of nursing education some good qualities may be discarded with the bad. A proper balance between academic training and practical experience should be the resolving factor. Both parties to the dispute should keep in mind the fact that bedside care will continue to be the major responsibility of most graduate nurses.

In the concerted attempt to shed the apron of apprenticeship we are apt to forget that nursing, like medicine, differs from most other vocations in one very vital respect – the nurse must put the interests of her patients above her own. Hours of work are immaterial when life is at stake. Dedication, self-discipline and a sense of personal responsibility are ingredients absolutely necessary to the development of a competent and trustworthy nurse. In recent years autonomous nursing schools, unaffiliated with hospitals, have sprung up in great numbers in the new community and technical colleges and the collèges d'enseignement général et professionel (CEGEPs) in Quebec. It will be up to these new schools to prove they are capable of producing this kind of dedicated graduate.

Some of these new schools, representatives of an emerging new kind of nursing education, offer straight two-year courses, others are of the 'two-plus-one' type. In 1970 there were 75 hospital schools of nursing, reduced from 171 a decade earlier. There were 70 regional and other schools of nursing. Of these 145 hospital and regional schools, about 40 were, or are about to become, two-year courses. It is interesting to note that in Quebec, where all the hospital schools have been phased out, CEGEP nursing courses are of three years duration.[4]

Although some nursing schools seem to be having second thoughts about the adequacy of preparation which the two-year course affords the new graduate, the trend to shorten the traditional three-year course seems to be continuing as we enter the seventies. At the same time some of the university schools of nursing are considering lengthening their courses to five years. In 1970 there were twenty-two university schools of nursing, all

4 The first year is basically a pre-selection year with a minimum of nursing content. The student then chooses a particular occupation in the health field for the second and third years.

but a few offering integrated programs leading to a baccalaureate degree. The computer age is with us and we hear murmurings of 'computerized nursing service.' Is it possible that the computer can replace the personal touch which has given confidence and care to the patients? In preparation for the so-called post-industrial society, represented by the computer, nurses across Canada have taken part in quantitative research in many areas of concern – work measurement, work activity, work distribution, patient dependency and nurse-patient ratio studies. From these analyses, nursing hours have been calculated, staffing requirements have been estimated and in a few hospitals the computer is recommending staffing patterns. More important, these studies have shown the need for more clear-cut delineation of the functions of nursing, not only those now assigned to graduate and auxiliary personnel, but also those in other hospital departments where there are areas of overlapping and confusion in the role of members of the health team. There seems to be an increasing awareness that the nursing service department must function not in isolation but as an integral part of the hospital. Administrative practices, policies and efficiency in the hospital as a whole are recognized as having deep-rooted implications for the administration of the nursing service within the overall administration of the hospital.

A glance into the crystal ball shows the nurse of the next half century as increasingly concerned with health as well as illness. She will have the knowledge and the skills to apply at the bedside, but she will also give thought to the patient's family, his community and the social and economic aspects of his illness. No longer will the nurse be confined to the 'do' of nursing but will as well be stimulated and encouraged to look outward and to enquire into the 'why.' The rigid discipline of the past is gone and today the nurse can look forward within her profession to a future of great opportunity, with the satisfaction of rewards – spiritual, mental and monetary – commensurate with her professional education and her patient responsibilities.

ADMINISTRATORS

The position of hospital superintendent has undergone considerable change over the last half century. For many years it was considered to be a position which, as one board chairman described it to me 'could be filled by anyone with a reasonable degree of intelligence.' It often seemed that way. The larger lay hospitals often appointed a man with no previous hospital experience and the practice is not entirely dead even today. I knew many of them well and they often told me how they learned the hard – and often bitter – way. Some were local businessmen, some were relatives of influential board members, some were retired bankers or businessmen, some were former army officers in need of a civilian job, some were former military medical officers preferring not to return to practice, some were civilian doctors wanting to forsake private practice. In the case of municipal hospitals, some supervisory positions were filled by former municipal employees or friends of civic office-holders.

In the smaller hospitals (and some large hospitals) the superintendent was often a nurse who had acquired some supervisory experience; several large non-religious hospitals have had nurse administrators, and a few still have but their number is decreasing. Sometimes, however, in a staff emergency, a graduate nurse with no administrative experience was named as acting superintendent and soon found herself with a permanent appointment. In Sisters' hospitals the custom of changing appointments every few years often resulted in an experienced Superior and superintendent being moved to a less responsible position and replaced by another Sister, probably competent as a Superior but quite inexperienced in hospital administration.

In the case of tuberculosis sanatoria the majority of superintendents were ex-patients, usually physicians who had recovered and realized that a career in sanatorium administration would be a wise choice. They, too, learned administration 'on the job.'

The personal devotion of these superintendents was noteworthy. Too often they worked under the handicaps of frustration, lack of assistants and a barrage of complaints from staff and community alike. By today's standards the hospital expected too much of its chief – and usually sole – executive. In smaller hospitals the superintendent (usually a nurse as already noted) was also head of the nursing services, purchasing agent, personnel officer, public relations officer, receiver of doctors' messages, enforcer of visiting regulations, custodian of the nurses' residence and opener of the morning mail. The only other person with as many duties was probably the one and only office worker, who had to be information clerk, bookkeeper, telephone operator, cashier, custodian of the medical records, payroll clerk, stenographer and general Pooh Bah. The smaller hospital could not supply any significant patient statistics or financial figures beyond those required for the rather superficial monthly statement, concerned mainly with the current cash position. It was not until the provincial governments began to require increasingly extensive patient and financial data that the present excellent statistical analyses were developed.

These comments are not to suggest that the hospitals were poorly administered. The spirit of dedication which seems to imbue all who work for hospitals must have been contagious; most of the superintendents of the day were conscientious and soon became enthusiastic about their work. They were generally intelligent individuals and quickly learned what should be done and what should not. Most problems could, and still can, be solved by common sense and a judicious application of diplomacy. The non-medical administrators sometimes had difficulty understanding the viewpoint of the medical staff, but they quickly learned that doctors are not difficult to lead but strenuously resist being pushed.

Some met their Waterloo when they attempted to restrict the authority of the director of nursing – especially if she was a martinet. She usually won and the administrator resigned.

Some took a while to realize that hospital administration is more than keeping out of the red and that quality of care is a *sine qua non*. The medically trained superintendent, on the other hand, usually knew little of accounting and of administrative principles, or of personnel management. He had to learn these skills on the job.

The interesting observation is that, despite this lack of training for the job and sometimes little or no previous experience of the chief executive, the hospitals were remarkably well managed. There was widespread loyalty among the personnel and a genuine pride in work – certainly much more than has been evident since hospital workers have been organized in unions.

Much credit, too, for the success of the hospitals over those years must be given to the board members. Selected for their altruistic interest and for the success of their personal careers, these men and women, serving without remuneration, have contributed more to their communities than will ever be realized. In many instances the chairman of the board, or the chairman of the finance or the house committee, has kept a 'new-broom' superintendent from making hasty or unfortunate decisions before he understood all the factors involved.

For many decades the position of the board and that of the superintendent had been clearly defined: the board initiated the policies and the superintendent carried them out. That is still the arrangement in most hospitals. But one can see the beginnings of a change in this arrangement, particularly in the United States. As new administrators come to their jobs with increasingly higher standards of training and experience, quite a few are assuming decision-making roles.

This change has been gradual but has been accelerating in the last decade. Boards need more expert guidance than ever before; men and women of board calibre are already carrying as much responsibility as they can and cannot be expected to become authorities in the many aspects of hospital activity. This means more reliance on the expert in their midst, the administrator; he, in turn, must depend upon his assistants for expert advice in their respective areas. The administrator is often now a consultant to his board in such matters as planning and the purchase of major equipment. A half century ago the superintendent of many large hospitals could not spend more than $200 on anything without board approval. In small hospitals the limit was often $25 and, to my knowledge, some hospitals imposed a ceiling that was not much higher until quite recently. In recent years, however, the administrator has been accorded more freedom. His judgment is respected and his latitude to act expanded.

Lines of authority are being more carefully delineated. The administrator of a hospital has been likened to the captain of a ship with full authority resting with him on the bridge. But the analogy has not always held and one does not need to go too far back to find examples. In some instances, the nursing service and the training school have been directly responsible to a special committee of the board, which frequently included members from the community at large – the local high school principal and nursing school alumnae, for example. Sooner or later this division of authority has led to confrontations. Sometimes a new administrator, thinking he truly had been appointed 'captain of the ship,' found that on the nursing floors and elsewhere he was, in fact, little more than the first mate's cabin boy.

A similar division of responsibility has occurred in the business office. The chairman of the finance committee (a board member) often has taken over direction of the accounts receivable and arranged collection procedures and handled presentations to municipal and county councils. This was more common in small hospitals where the nurse-superintendent directed the patient-service aspects of the daily tasks and was happy to leave financial matters to the businessmen on the board. In the union hospitals on the Prairies one of the municipal officers is chief executive of the hospital and this arrangement has produced some excellent administrators of hospitals as well as some first-rate officers of the hospital associations.

Sometimes the splitting off of financial responsibility from general administration has been carried too far. It is one thing for the administrator to be relieved of financial responsibility; it is quite another matter for him to be kept unaware of his hospital's financial situation, as sometimes used to happen. As late as the 1950s in one medium-sized hospital, a new well-qualified administrator found that his accountant was forbidden, under any circumstance, to show the administrator the monthly financial statement before it had been presented to the board. This order from the chairman of the finance committee put the administrator in an untenable position, not only with respect to intelligent operation of his hospital but by denying him authority over his subordinates. The administrator naturally left for another hospital where he could function properly.

Today the lines of authority are becoming more clearly defined. In a number of our larger hospitals, the former administrator now has become the 'executive director.' This was accomplished by a re-definition and expansion of the duties involved, with more emphasis on leadership qualities. An administrator and one or more assistant administrators are then responsible to him. They, in turn, have specific responsibilities for various departments in the hospital.

This gives him more time to develop policies for submission to the board and also to deal with the various bodies and agencies which are concerned with the care of the patient and the operation of the hospital.

This increased status has led to another development. Traditionally the superintendent was the paid servant of the board, whose desires and decisions he implemented. Now, more than ever, he sits on the board, not on invitation but by right, as an essential advisor. He participates freely in discussions of hospital policy and direction.

This situation has raised the question, 'Should the hospital administrator (executive director) sit as a member of the board?' It seems contrary to the long-established practice of thinking of the administrator as a salaried employee only. The arrangement is common in business however, where corporate officers are often board members as well. Hospital boards are accepting this arrangement in increasing numbers and a number of administrators are being made 'executive vice-president' of their hospital. In fact, in a number of large u.s. hospitals, the board has gone the whole way and made the administrator or executive director the president of the hospital. Sometimes he is termed president and managing director. This is an acknowledgement of the worth of a well-qualified and experienced administrator. Still, it does cast the trustee into a more shadowy role and denies him a degree of public recognition for the tremendous amount of donated service he gives the board.

Whether the administrator sitting on the board should vote on issues confronting the trustees is a debatable point. It can be argued that his vote would most likely be an intelligent one on the issue involved; moreover, it would more certainly commit him to prompt and supportive executive action. As a board member he might find it easier to get support for his own proposals.

However, from the viewpoint of his own protection and his effectiveness as a neutral administrator of board policy, there is a distinct element of danger if he 'takes sides' in voting. Sometimes issues can arouse quite violent emotions and he could find himself voting with the minority group. This could cause the majority to question his judgment and perhaps shake their confidence in him. This puts a senior employee into a position fraught with potential danger. In some respects his post is analogous to that of a deputy minister when there is a change of government – except that the hospital administrator lacks the tenured protection of the civil servant.

In summary, between 1920 and 1970 the status of the hospital superintendent has climbed from administrator to executive director, to executive vice-president and now to president. We should add, however, that the great majority are still administrators and attend – but not as voting members – the meetings of the board. Under any terminology, it is a far cry from the days of the monastic hospitals in medieval Europe when the 'warden' could not leave the hospital, or, if permitted to leave, he could not wander more than a mile or so; he could not visit the alehouse, nor could he play cards, roll dice, or play handball. Apparently he had one outlet for self-expression – he was permitted to discipline the staff or the patients as he saw fit.

The increased status of hospital administrators is the result of the ever-increasing qualifications and management expertise demanded to run today's complex hospitals.

During the twenties there were no formal training courses for administrators and few opportunities for the hospital superintendents to exchange ideas. A few provincial or regional hospital associations were being formed but they were operating on a shoestring and did not have much activity apart from annual meetings. There was no national organization or service in Canada before the Canadian Medical Association's Department of Hospital Service was formed in 1928. A few progressive hospitals were members of the American Hospital Association with its lending library and quite a few subscribed to the American hospital journals, notably *Modern Hospital, Hospital Management* and the journal of the Catholic Hospital Association, *Hospital Progress*. The publication of the American Hospital Association was still a small quarterly and did not become the monthly (now bi-weekly) *Hospitals* until the mid-thirties. *The Canadian Hospital* was launched in 1924 and was much more tailored to Canadian needs.

During the 1920s an increasing number of Canadian superintendents, more than were members, attended the annual convention of the American Hospital Association, always a very rewarding experience. In the late 1920s and 1930s the standardization conference held in conjunction with the winter convention of the American College of Surgeons provided a varied program of hospital topics and proved to be another most stimulating gathering. However, institutes and refresher courses were not available.

Dr MacEachern's comprehensive text book, *Hospital Organization and Management*, for many years the bible of the administrator, was published in 1935. This was soon on the desk of every progressive hospital administrator. Meanwhile the requirements for full approval under the standardization of the American College of Surgeons, so ably and personally directed by Dr MacEachern, was giving the hospital boards and administration an idea of what should be the objectives of every good hospital and its medical staff. A few years later, in 1939, Dr Thomas R. Ponton's book, *The Medical Staff in the Hospital*, came out and made a noticeable impression on staff organization and relationships.

Influence of the American College of Hospital Administrators
When the American College of Hospital Administrators was formed in 1933, few of that small group could have realized how rapidly it would grow or how influential it would become.

For some time Dr Malcolm MacEachern had been stressing the need for a professional appraising body. Matthew Foley, editor of *Hospital Management*, supported the idea in his columns. Impatient with the slow progress of the idea, Matt Foley went to Dewey Lutes, then president of the Chicago and Illinois Hospital Association, and asked him to set up an organizing committee. Lutes did as Foley asked and the college was constituted with Charles Wordell as president and Dewey Lutes as director-general. A number of Canadians and former Canadians were invited to beome charter fellows; some Canadians not directing hospitals were invited to join as honorary fellows.

This body, like the standardization movement, encountered not only apathy but downright opposition from some of the leading administrators who felt that it was just another status-seeking group. Indeed, in the early days, this attitude might have had some justification, for those of us on the supposedly anonymous credentials committee under the chairmanship of Dr MacEachern were deluged with applications of questionable merit. In the early days, some applicants were awarded fellowships with little evidence of outstanding merit other than thirty or more years of continous service. (Of course, that, in itself, may have been sufficient to warrant recognition.) Rising standards for qualification and the many achievements of the college have long since removed the early doubts. Through its regional institutes, publications, examinations and annual meetings the college has been a major factor in the stimulation of greater qualification in the administrative field. Incidentally, with the setting up of the college, the hospital superintendents from that time on became 'administrators,' actually a much more appropriate term.

Many Canadians have served on the board of governors and on the council of regents of the ACHA and two have been presidents – Arthur J. Swanson of the Toronto Western Hospital for 1956–7 and Dr Arnold L Swanson, then of the Victoria General Hospital in London, Ontario, for 1969–70.

Graduate Training in Hospital Administration
The next step in the evolution of the administrator was the establishment of formal training courses. It was obvious that the administration of a hospital with its increasing complexity of detail required an executive who had more than the *ordinary* knowledge of administrative principles, of human relations, of medical problems, of socio-economic developments, of business procedures, of medico-legal dangers, of pedagogic methods and of the importance of public relations.

Credit for the first graduate course goes to Marquette University, which established one in 1928. It was discontinued the following year because of lack of enrolment. However, other universities and individuals were becoming interested. One pioneer was Michal Davis, PH D who had long been interested in cost and other studies in the health field. Davis was director of the Rosenwald Foundation and was playing an active role in developing the Councils of the American Hospital Association. With assistance from the Commonwealth Fund he set up a graduate course in hospital administration at the University of Chicago in 1934 with Dr Arthur Bachmeyer as director (and director of the University of Chicago Clinics until his untimely death in 1953). This course set a new standard in the training of administrators. Three years later, 1937, an undergraduate course was started at St Louis University, designed primarily for Catholic Sisters seeking greater proficiency in administrative techniques. In 1948 the course became a graduate one. Northwestern University in Chicago set up a course in 1943 with the financial help of the Johnson and Johnson Research Foundation and the American Hospital Supply Corporation. Dr M.T. MacEachern was director and Miss Laura Jackson was his assistant. An innovation at Northwestern was the introduction of evening classes which permitted many of the students to gain practical experience during the day (not to mention the necessary wherewithal) while obtaining their degrees.

At this time the W.K. Kellogg Foundation gave a tremendous impetus to education in hospital administration. The foundation underwrote the initial years of courses at Columbia, Johns Hopkins (since discontinued), Yale, Washington University at St Louis and Minnesota.

No courses had been started as yet in Canada. In 1947, Graham Davis, who was in charge of the hospital field programs of the Kellogg Foundation, offered assistance to the University of Toronto to establish a course in hospital administration. This course was set up in the school of public health (as were the courses at Columbia, Minnesota and Yale) in order to encourage a closer relationship between public health and the clinical aspects of health care. Such a close linkage, it was hoped, would overcome the polarization so prevalent on this continent.

The Kellogg offer of financial assistance was accepted by the University of Toronto and in 1947 a graduate course was started in the School of Hygiene under my direction. Dr L.O. Bradley who had recently taken his hospital administration degree at the university of Chicago was a full-time associate for the first three years. In 1948 we were joined by Eugenie Stuart, a nurse with considerable administration experience in Canada and South Africa and a graduate of MacEachern's course in hospital administration at Northwestern. She was mother confessor to succeeding classes for more than twenty years until her retirement in 1971.

The course required a baccalaureate for admission and consisted of one academic year of eight to nine months work on the campus with frequent field trips to hospitals and health agencies followed by a residency of twelve months in a selected hospital where the administrator-preceptor would prescribe a rotating schedule and work assignments for the resident. In later years the allocations were confined to hospitals within reasonable driving distance of Toronto so that the second-year students could participate in on-campus seminars every second week. Before graduation, each student was required to write a major dissertation or thesis. Since 1962 Dr Burns Roth, a graduate of the course and former deputy minister of health in Saskatchewan, has been in charge.

Other Canadian courses followed. An excellent program was developed at the University of Montreal. Its first director was Dr Gerald Lasalle, a graduate in medicine of Laval and in hospital administration of Toronto. The Montreal course was inaugurated in 1956 and included nine months' academic work and a year of residency. When Dr Lasalle went to Sherbrooke, first as dean of the new medical school, then as vice-rector of the university, Dr Gilbert Blain became the course director. Recently the course has been changed to provide two eight-month academic years with a four-month residency between and an eight-month residency at the end – 28 months in all. This appears to be an excellent solution to the problem of integrating academic and practical training. It is anticipated that this will result in a more thorough training in financial administration and a better knowledge of the problems of medical care administration.

In 1964, Rev A.L.M. Danis, executive director of the Catholic Hospital Association of Canada, set up and became director of the graduate school of hospital administration at the University of Ottawa. The Ottawa program is traditional but with a stronger-than-usual emphasis on a knowledge of the health environment as a whole, rather than on institutional management. An interesting experiment in group residency rotating among hospitals has been introduced. Some of the students have served their residency with a regional hospital planning council. Instruction in the Ottawa course is largely in English but the course does have the advantage of operating in what is essentially a bilingual environment.

The latest course was developed by the University of Alberta under the direction of Carl A. Meilike, a graduate of the University of Toronto course, with the assistance of the W.K. Kellogg Foundation. A progressive feature of the Alberta course is that the faculty designs individual courses for each student according to his needs and objectives. (*All* courses do that to some degree; for example, a physician would not require medical orientation and a student with a bachelor's degree in business administration would not need to repeat accounting.) However, the Alberta course is unique in custom-tailoring each course to the student's planned career.

In the 1960s the University of Saskatchewan offered a graduate course in business administration with an option in health-care administration. This option was discontinued in 1968 as the comprehensive health program developed at the University of Alberta. However, Saskatchewan has continued with a two year correspondence course, designed primarily for those already involved in the administration of small and medium-sized hospitals. It is under the supervision of Frank H. Silversides.

The University of British Columbia developed an undergraduate program in 1952. This was a six-and-one-half year course, including eighteen months in residency. Graduates were awarded a bachelor of commerce degree and a diploma in hospital administration. The UBC course was unique; the students in the School of Commerce had to have some prior knowledge of hospitals and had to be known as suitable by the dean, Professor E.D. MacPhee. In their third year the students could choose the option in hospital administration. If approved by the dean they served four months as summer relief at the Vancouver General Hospital which required the approval of the executive director, Leon Hickernell. Classes proved to be small despite a good curriculum, and in 1957 the course was discontinued.

In September 1971, the University of British Columbia set up a Department of Health Care and Epidemiology with a heavy emphasis on research. Only those with considerable training and experience in health service will be active in this new program.

Courses in Health Administration

As the summaries above show, the trend in university courses in hospital administration is towards a broadening of content. In recent years it has become apparent that the various aspects of the overall health program are becoming more closely related. Only part of the work of public health departments relates to epidemic control, water treatment, sewage disposal and so on. The fundamental tenets of society have come under scrutiny and the development of tax-supported health insurance has opened up the need for executives trained in that particular phase of administration. Actually, many of the graduates of the university courses in hospital administration are now employed in provincial and federal health departments. Others work in health insurance programs or hospital and medical association offices. It is obvious that there is now a need for individuals trained in *health* administration, of which *hospital* administration would be a major segment. Columbia was one of the first to emphasize the wider concept and other universities have broadened their courses also.

The University of Toronto, recognizing the need for a more comprehensive course, overhauled the curriculum and placed the course under the renamed Department of Health Administration in the late sixties. The University of Montreal incorporates this broader training, including medical care administration in its lengthened course.

These modifications, broadening the base of study, should prove beneficial provided the necessity of giving future hospital administrators a sound preparation to meet the specific and increasing problems of hospitals is not lost in a confusion of options and alternatives.

The university programs have benefited from the Association of University Programs in Hospital Administration, set up in 1948 to assess and to provide standards by which courses could be evaluated. Starting with a handful of charter members, of which Toronto was the only Canadian, there are now more than thirty graduate courses approved and others under consideration. The association requires any new program applying for recognition to have been in operation at least one year. Teams of evaluators visit the schools administering the courses at regular intervals. Courses are encouraged to experiment with new approaches, but each must conform to an accepted basis of educational content and procedure. Courses developed in schools of public health (Toronto is an example) must also meet the approval of the American Public Health Association.

For those who helped develop these various courses in hospital and health administration, there has been an immense degree of personal happiness. In a very real sense, the teacher lives on through his students' accomplishments. For twenty-five years and more, those of us who have taught in the courses have taken endless pride in the graduates who go out and shoulder responsibilities quickly and competently. Many, although still quite young in years, have already assumed some of the toughest administrative assignments on this continent. Others hold high national or regional positions and some have already had high honours conferred upon them.[5]

Extension Courses
Even as the American and Canadian colleges set up their courses in hospital administration, it was recognized they could never graduate enough students to fill the need. There are more than eight thousand approved or registered hospitals in the two countries; it would take years and years before all the graduate courses combined could produce *that* number of graduates. Additionally, many of the larger hospitals required not one graduate but two or three more as the chief's deputies. Still further, not all graduates went to work in hospitals; many took positions in government health departments, others in the various health and hospital associations. Non-course graduates, it was realized, would be serving as hospital administrators for years to come. How could they be helped to up-grade their qualifications?

In 1950 Dr L.O. Bradley, then secretary of the Canadian Hospital Council, suggested that the non-graduate administrators should be provided with a course, too. Fraser Armstrong, president of the CHC, agreed and the following year a committee on education was set up with myself as chairman, Rev Hector Bertrand as vice-chairman and Dr Bradley as secretary. Graham Davis of the Kellogg Foundation was approached. Davis approved

5 For instance, Dr George W. Graham, a graduate in medicine of McGill (1941) and of Toronto in hospital administration (1950) was president of the American Hospital Association in 1969.

of the scheme but felt the course would be most effective if it had a university connection. Dr R.D. Defries, director of the School of Hygiene at the University of Toronto, Dr William J. Dunlop, director of that university's extension programs and President Sidney E. Smith approved the relationship. The Department of Hospital Administration agreed to oversee the preparation of lessons with Donald M. MacIntyre (later the administrator of the Kingston General Hospital) in charge. The text, prepared by many collaborators, is an unexcelled compilation of what an administrator needs to know. The Kellogg Foundation agreed to provide $110,000 to underwrite the first few years and the extension course in hospital organization and management was under way.

This course of thirty home lessons and three weeks each summer for two years was designed primarily for those administrators (or senior staff of administrator potential) who did not have a bachelor's degree and were, therefore, barred from the graduate courses. Because of the tremendous demand for inclusion (and with classes limited to 150), each province was given a proportionate quota, the selection to be made by the provincial hospital association. The first summer course was held at Queen's University at Kingston, Ontario, in 1952. During more recent years it has been held at the University of Manitoba, a central and very suitable location, which will probably be its permanent location.

From the completion of the first course to 1970, this course issued certificates to more than fourteen hundred men and women, no mean achievement.

In 1948 Father Hector Bertrand and other hospital leaders in Quebec set up a series of workshops on all phases of hospital activity. Although not solely for administrators they were exceptionally valuable for those administrative personnel who attended. In 1954 these workshops were organized into a course for which recognition was given upon completion. Father Bertrand and Roland Levert were satisfied with nothing less than the highest standards of the course; hospital experts from across the continent were consulted about each workshop. When qualified French-speaking instructors were unavailable, English-speaking experts delivered the lectures with translation supplied. A valuable service was provided to thousands of hospital workers in Quebec throughout the 1950s. Since the early sixties when the activities of le Comité des Hôpitaux were phased out, the University of Montreal and the Canadian Hospital Association course in hospital organization and management have attempted to fill the gap.

Administrators' Associations in Canada
In the past fifteen years four provinical administrators' associations have been organized, in Quebec, British Columbia, Saskatchewan and Nova Scotia. All have served as valuable forums for the exchange of ideas on developing trends in hospital administration. In Quebec, l'Association des Administrateurs d'Hôpitaux has published *L'Hôpital d'aujourd'hui* since the early 1960s.

The Canadian College of Health Service Executives
This lusty young infant came into being at the 1970 convention of the Canadian Hospital Association in Edmonton. Its gestation period had been lengthy, dating back over a decade to a meeting in British Columbia of some of the administrators attending the Western Canada Institute. The desire for such an association was encouraged by the many graduates of the university courses and of the extension course of the Canadian Hospital Association – by all administrative personnel who sought a continuing avenue of education. Also there were some who found the increasingly exacting standards of the American College of Hospital Administrators a frustrating hurdle.

After a careful study of the situation by a committee of the Canadian Hospital Association under the chairmanship of Dr Douglas Wallace (then executive director of the Toronto General Hospital and later executive director of the Canadian Medical Association), the CHA sponsored in 1970 the creation of what was, at first, called the Canadian Council of Hospital Administrators. Following the Edmonton meeting in 1970, the body's membership and function was broadened and the organization was renamed the Canadian Council of Health Service Executives. At the 1971 meeting in Montreal the name was again changed to the Canadian College of Health Service Executives. The first president was Dr L.O. Bradley. Other members of the first executive are listed in Appendix I. Membership has grown rapidly to more than five hundred at the time of writing. Eligibility for participation has been made sufficiently broad to cover individuals holding executive positions of responsiblity in the health field and advancement is by prescribed avenues of achievement. The by-laws provide for three levels of membership – affiliate, associate and active. Active membership requires the applicant to hold a post of senior management responsibility acceptable to the credentials committee and to have had tenure of at least five years. He must also have accumulated fifty credits. These credits are given for the holding of a graduate diploma or degree in hospital administration or public health; a baccalaureate; service in years; par-

ticipation in the work of national, provincial or other specified areas in the
health field; publications; and educational contibutions. The creation of a
fellowship category will probably follow.[6] But the college is rightly taking
time to ensure that the standard required will be in keeping with its lofty
objectives.

There is every indication that the college will complement, rather than
be in competition with, the American College of Hospital Administrators.
Many of its charter members are also members or fellows of the ACHA. The
latter will continue to draw membership in Canada and will continue to provide educational programs to its members and fellows, but the Canadian
college will provide educational facilities to a broader group of health service executives, irrespective of educational background, and should be
able to more effectively help those most needing the stimulus of educational opportunity.

A Code of Ethics for Administrators and Their Hospitals
For twenty-four centuries the medical profession has had a rigid code of
ethics in the Oath of Hippocrates which has been revised from time to time
to meet changing conditions. Nurses have followed several principles of
ethics and adopted the code formulated by the International Council of
Nurses in the early 1950s. Various paramedical personnel have observed
the necessity of keeping records and the results of tests and procedures
confidential.

However for many years there was no general ethical code applicable
to all hospitals and to all personnel. At the same time, such a code was emi-
nently desirable, especially with respect to the administrator. In his key
position ethical practices were most essential if staff morale and public confidence were to be maintained. Dr Malcom MacEachern stressed this need
continually.

The 'last straw' which led to the creation of such a code may have been
the actions of some of the younger administrators who, craving instant recognition, endorsed some new piece of equipment in extravagant language.
The hastily written testimonial, complete with the inevitable protrait of its
author, appeared in the advertising pages of the journals in due course. The
American College of Hospital Administrators set up a committee in 1938
to study the whole subject of ethics and, if desired, to draft such a code.
Through their membership in the ACHA, Canadian administrators became
interested in the study. Presumably on the theory that it takes a thief to

6 Dr Agnew was made the first honorary fellow at the 1971 meeting in Montreal.

catch a thief, I was asked to chair the committee; fortunately the other members could not have been more carefully chosen. It did not take the committee long to realize that there could not be a code for administrators only; all personnel should be covered. Accordingly, the American Hospital Association, to which a large proportion of larger Canadian hospitals belonged, made it a joint undertaking and named the same committee to represent it as well.

The study committee encountered diverse views. While the great majority of comments received were commendatory with repeated admonitions to 'make it tough,' there were some who questioned the need of any code. 'If you're a gentleman, you don't need any code; if you're not, you won't observe it anyway.' Or, the old cliché, 'You can't make a silk purse out of a sow's ear.'

Well, you *can* make silk out of wood, coal and dear knows what, so maybe it could be done. (In fact, chemists have told me that one of their profession actually *did* transform the sow's ear.) Since it is a fact that hospital administrators and other staff in these countries do come from countries on every continent, many of them with widely differing concepts of business and personal relationships, the committee concluded that a code of ethics was definitely needed. One was prepared, presented and adopted in 1941. The code was also adopted by the Canadian Hospital Council in 1941 and approved in principle by the Canadian Medical Association.

Catholic Hospitals
A code of ethics for Catholic hospitals was first formulated in 1919 by Rev Charles B. Moulinier, sj, the founder of the Catholic Hospital Association of the United States and Canada. It was somewhat limited as it dealt primarily with certain surgical and obstetrical practices. At about this period several of the Catholic dioceses prepared their own, broader codes for the guidance of their hospitals. One frequently used in other areas was that of the Diocese of Hartford. A book, *Ethics of Ectopic Operations* by Rev Timothy L. Bouscaren, sj (published by Loyola University Press) in the 1930s provided a widely accepted interpretation which was considerably less severe than those advanced earlier by Antonelli, Noldin-Schmidtt, Sabetti-Barrett and others. Father Gerald Kely, sj, wrote frequently on ethics in *Hospital Progress, The Linacre Quarterly*, and other journals. In 1949, Rev Alphonse M. Schwitalla, president of the Catholic Hospital Association of the United States and Canada published 'Ethical and Religious Directives for Catholic Hospitals.' This became the basis for

the American 'Code of Ethics for Catholic Hospitals' published in chart and pamphlet form in 1954 and the 'Moral Code' published at that time by the Catholic Hospital Association of Canada, available in both English and French. The 'Ethical and Religious Directives,' by the way, is not in itself an official code in any diocese unless the bishop adopts it.

These 'Ethical Directives' have been clearly expressed and have proven of great help not only to the medical and lay staffs of the Catholic hospitals but to others as well. I have discussed them at length with graduate classes in hopital administration, with extension classes and with various hospital and medical groups, for it is important that the administrative and medical staffs of non-Catholic hospitals understand why the Catholic hospitals follow, or do not follow, certain procedures.

While, as the directives point out, the principles do not change, some interpretations have undergone change. There seems to be more priority placed upon preserving the mother's life today than in the interpretation we received as medical students. Recent liberalization of abortion laws in Canada and the setting up of abortion committees have created new procedural decisions for the Sister Superior and her council. The problems, as we move into the seventies, seem to be resolving satisfactorily, particularly where a non-Catholic hospital is in the area.

Changing Form of Administration in Sisters' Hospitals
During the 1950s and 1960s an increasing number of lay administrators were appointed in the Sisters' hospitals. Earlier, the Sister Superior usually served as administrator as well. However, administration steadily was becoming a more complex task, not entirely compatible with the prevailing practice of shifting a sister's duties and, often, her location, every few years. This may have been democratic and preserved humility in the individual but it often meant a loss to the hospital and frequently to the entire region, when the Sister who was moved had gained administrative experience. After the second world war I began to note an increasing number of lay business managers as well. Also, I noted, in working with a number of the hospitals, the local lay advisory boards were being given more executive power with respect to finance, expansion and personnel relations. In the 1960s, particularly, a number of the Sisters' hospitals appointed well-qualified lay administrators. Matters of ethics, religious observances and related concern still came under the Sister Superior and her sisters' council. It should be noted, however, that the great majority of administrators in Sisters' hospitals are still members of the order.

Licensure of Administrators
It has sometimes been said (in hospital circles) that the only workers who did not require some form of license or approval were the maids and the administrators. An exaggeration, of course, but it is becoming more obvious with each decade that more and more classes of employees holding positions of responsibility are being subject to some form of approval. In some cases the approval is granted by governmental fiat and is, therefore, mandatory. In other cases the approval is granted by various bodies or organizations representing certain specific interests within the hospital. Although not compelled by law to obtain approval from these semi-official bodies, nevertheless if the hospital wishes to operate in the field in which the approval-granting organization is recognized, it is under great pressure to obtain approval for its personnel in that area of work.

Licensure of administrators was initiated some years ago in the United States by the State of Minnesota. While not too disturbing of the status quo it did require increasing standards of experience and/or training for the post of administrator in the more responsible positions.

Until today, licensing of administrators had not been adopted in any Canadian province or any other state. In the forties, Saskatchewan was interested and the government actually drafted a bill which did not carry when it was realized that it would make it difficult for the Sisters to continue their rotation system.

It seems surprising that there has not been more effort to bring about licensure for administration, considering the responsibility of the position and the extensive qualities required.

The membership and fellowship of the American College of Hospital Administrators, the hospital organization and management extension course of the Canadian Hospital Association and the postgraduate, two-year courses in hospital administration given by several universities, have helped to raise the qualifications of administrators. The Canadian College of Health Service Executives intends to add to these efforts in the years ahead.

Conclusion
Hospitals are infinitely better managed now than ever before. We can derive great satisfaction from the progressive and conscientious service given to the public by those who bear the responsibility of hospital management. During the seventies I believe administration must assume a greater role than that of maintaining a well-operated hospital. It is not enough to do the work that presents itself daily – to keep the hospital up to date, to

preserve good public relations and to do one's share of committee and other work for the provincial and national associations. The whole health field is undergoing tremendous change in scientific progress, in medico-economics, in welfare methods, in labor relations, in methods of medical practice, in hospital finance and in public health relations. The hospitals are involved in practically all of them.

We must have administrators whose breadth of vision is sufficient to encompass all of the problems, administrators who can see the possibilities ahead and who can help lead the way. If the hospital is to attain its full potential and meet its obligation it must be led into a broadened concept of its function in the local, provincial and national health programs. This involves a greater appreciation of the possible roles of our hospitals, not only in the care of the patient, in education and in research (the time-honored trinity of objectives) but with respect to the many other facets of community health programs, the changing relationships to the medical profession and the changing application of social welfare concepts.

OTHER HOSPITAL PERSONNEL

In 1970, there were more than one hundred different job classifications for hospital personnel in large urban hospitals. Some of these classifications reflect increasing educational and research activities. Others simply demonstrate the enormous growth in the volume and variety of patient services. Perhaps the best indicator of the increasing complexity of diagnosis and therapy has been the rapid development of the paramedical occupations.

Paramedicals
Generated by a labor-intensive medical technology, paramedical workers have facilitated a higher standard of patient care and a more efficient utilization of medical manpower. Laboratory technologists, radiological technicians, physical and occupational therapists, inhalation therapy technicians, electroencephalography technicians, medical electronics technicians and others are needed for their therapeutic or technical skills. Medical record librarians, dietitians and others also provide specialized services which promote greater efficiency and quality care.

The greatest impetus to better and more standardized qualifications among paramedicals has come from occupational societies and associations. In many cases these societies, often with the co-operation and assistance of the Canadian Medical Association, established standards of approval for the training courses and set up annual examinations and other criteria for determining association membership or certification. Because licensure has generally not been required for paramedicals, the marks of recognition and expertise set up by the societies are crucial in assisting hospitals to judge the qualifications of paramedical personnel.

By far the three most prominent groups of paramedical workers based almost entirely within the hospital have been laboratory technologists, radiological technicians and medical record librarians.

Laboratory technologists
Probably the first acknowledged occasion of a need for trained assistants in the medical laboratory occurred during the emergency conditions of the first world war. During the 1920s laboratory workers hired by hospitals usually had no previous formal education in biochemistry or microbiology. The pathologist or other physicians who worked in the laboratory instructed the new assistants in routine procedures and a few basic laws of chemistry. It was a practical approach and produced some good technologists. Unfortunately the system also produced some who weren't so good and a need to standardize the instruction of lab technologists became apparent. Under the encouragement of the American College of Surgeons' standardization program (and the sponsorship of the American Society of Clinical Pathologists) the American Registry of Medical Technologists was set up in 1928. As there was no similar organization in Canada until 1937, the Canadian graduates who qualified initially registered with the American body.

Late in 1936 three laboratory technologists at the Hamilton General Hospital decided to organize a national society with the following objectives:

1 To improve the qualifications and standing of laboratory technicians in Canada.
2 To promote research endeavor in all branches of laboratory work.
3 To promote a recognized professional status for laboratory technicians in Canada.
4 To promote closer co-operation between the medical profession and the technician.
5 To more efficiently aid in diagnosing and treating disease.[7]

Frank J. Elliott was elected the first president of the Canadian Society of

7 From the charter of incorporation, May 1937

Laboratory Technologists (CSLT) and continued in that capacity until 1939. Dr W.J. Deadman and Ileen Kemp (now Mrs E. Parker) were active in the first years as a director and secretary respectively. Mrs Parker became society president in the late forties and served as its first full-time executive secretary from 1950 to 1961.

Two important functions of the society started in 1938 were the publication of *The Canadian Journal of Medical Technology* and the annual examinations for certification. An official registry was set up the following year with approval of the CMA. Under my chairmanship the Canadian Medical Association set up a special committee on approval of hospital laboratories for the training of laboratory technologists. The first list of approved laboratories showed ten institutions in four provinces. Over the years the CSLT became increasingly involved in the approval of these training laboratories and in 1969 joined with the CMA approvals committee in assessing qualified laboratories. The early training took place completely within the laboratory but during the sixties an increasing proportion of students took the first phase of their course in an academic setting such as a college of applied arts and technology.

The CSLT has branches or affiliated societies in all provinces. By 1970 membership in the national organization had reached 10,825.

Over the years the amount of work done in the laboratory has increased tremendously. Studies have shown that the number of laboratory tests doubled between 1925 and 1945; between 1945 and 1970 they increased more than fifteenfold. Some larger hospitals are currently doing more than a million tests annually. Not only has the quantity of tests grown enormously but so has their complexity. Specialization in laboratory technology has come into its own during the past decade in such areas as virology, hematology, parasitology and histology.

Radiological technicians
In 1895 William Roentgen discovered the mysterious form of radiant energy which he called the X-ray. Over the next twenty-five years tremendous accomplishments were made in adapting this energy for medical purposes. The hot-cathode vacuum tube and the nitrate-base X-ray film were two key developments which facilitated the widespread use of X-ray equipment in hospitals by 1920.

The first technicians were trained to handle films and care for equipment in military hospitals during the first world war. In the early 1920s the Radiological Society of North America and the American Roentgen Ray

Society set up a registry for X-ray technicians. Many Canadians were registered by this American Registry of Radiological Technicians.[8] There was no Canadian association before 1929, when the Western Society of Radiographers[9] was organized in Winnipeg. The Ontario Society of Radiographers, formed in 1935, took steps in the late 1930s to bring about the formation of associations for X-ray technicians in the other provinces (except for Manitoba where one already existed) as a preliminary step to a national federation. In 1942 the provincial societies in co-operation with the Canadian Medical Association and Candian Association of Radiologists formed the Canadian Society of Radiological Technicians. At the end of 1943 active membership was 386. Claude J. Bodle of Winnipeg was the first president.

The prime function of the society has been to improve the qualifications of technicians by holding registration examinations for graduates of approved two-year courses in radiologic technique. Curriculum standards were set up and after extensive negotiation with the Canadian Medical Association and the Canadian Association of Radiology, a joint committee on technical training was established in 1959.

The society's excellent journal *Focal Spot*, originally founded as the *Ontario Radiographer* in 1939, became the national publication four years later.

Medical record librarians
There was a great dearth of facilities for the training of medical record librarians in Canada during the early part of the 1920 to 1970 period. Only the better organized hospitals had medical record librarians prior to the first world war. The impetus to bring the clinical records department under a trained director (rather than under a committee of the medical staff) came to most hospitals under the stimulus of the ACS standardization program. More hospitals failed to gain approval because of inadequate or incomplete medical records than for any other reason.

For a long time there were only two schools for medical record librarians in Canada – that at St Michael's Hospital in Toronto, set up in 1936 by Sister Mary Paul, and that at the Hôtel Dieu in Kingston under Sister Campion, organized a few months later. In the early fifties others followed. By 1970 there were eleven medical record librarian schools in Canada; eight were located in hospitals, two in vocational schools and one in a university

8 In 1936 the name was changed to the American Registry of X-ray Technicians.
9 In 1940 it became the Manitoba Society of X-ray Technicians.

(at Notre Dame University, in Nelson, British Columbia). Basic requirements have been senior matriculation, a registered nurse's diploma, a teaching certificate or 12 months library experience in an approved hospital together with typing ability.

The first medical record librarians association formed was in Ontario with the encouragement of the Ontario Hospital Association. In 1935 five women representing five hospitals held an organizational meeting. Isabel Marshall of the Brantford General Hospital was the first president, assisted by Lillian Johnstone of the Hamilton General Hospital, who went on to serve the association for many years.

The Canadian Association of Medical Record Librarians (CAMRL) was formed in 1942. This was really a development of the earlier Ontario Medical Record Librarians Association. Various provincial associations have been formed since that time, functioning as regional branches of CAMRL. Annual meetings have increased in importance and have been addressed by outstanding speakers. The 1970 meeting was attended by 142 registrants.

In 1953 the Canadian Hospital Association in co-operation with CAMRL set up an extension course designed primarily for the large numbers of individuals, unqualified as medical record librarians, who were maintaining the medical records of smaller and, in some instances, fairly large hospitals. The hospital courses leading to registration were limited in their numbers of graduates and simply could not meet the needs of the more than 1,200 public and federal hospitals across Canada. Supported at first by the Kellogg Foundation, the extension course accepted applicants who were employed in a medical records library for the duration of the two-year course, four months of which was spent in a session actively supervised by a qualified instructor. A certificate was awarded on completion.

By 1962 CAMRL felt that the increased number of schools leading to registration would meet the needs of the larger hospitals and withdrew from this jointly sponsored course. However, there was still a marked shortage of medical record personnel in the smaller hospitals, so a revised extension program was planned for the technical level. From 1962 to 1970 some 364 medical record clerks and 419 technicians graduated from this course.

Summary
One of the unfortunate side effects of these drives for higher qualifications has been that too many people have put the emphasis on acquiring credentials rather than getting the job done. Many societies, associations and licensing bodies have made study requirements that seem unnecessary or

a waste of valuable time to the students; some of the unrest on university campuses undoubtedly has been due to this factor. Sometimes it has seemed that the objective was to maintain a short supply of paramedical workers. Most new societies have had fairly easy requirements for charter membership; and then standards are substantially raised over the years for new members – standards so exacting that many members of long standing could not meet them.

In the hospital field there has been considerable concern over the problems of overspecialization and fractionalization brought on by certification and licensure. There is a tremendous range of categories of health personnel, and the problem is to facilitate more flexibility in function in the light of our constant shortage of skilled manpower yet provide the safety to patients which is paramount.

Efforts to educate students about the roles and functions of other members of the health team, by contact in common classes, or by more formal means, are important. Medical, nursing, paramedical, administrative and other personnel must be continually aware of the overall objectives of the team and try to keep as broad a perspective as possible.

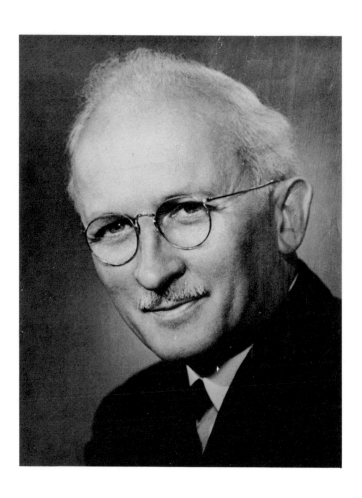

G. Harvey Agnew, MD, LLD, FACP, FACHA
1895–1971

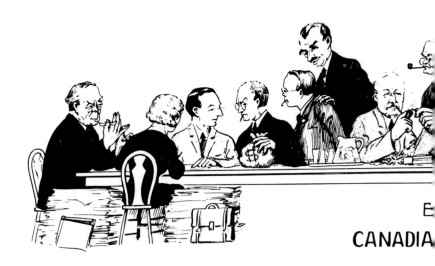

E
CANADIA

The executive committee of the Canadian Medical Association, 1931–2, depicted by Dr Agnew (who has anonymously fitted himself in, third from the right). From the left: A.T. Bazin, Mrs M. Campbell, T.C. Routley, F.S. Patch, A.S. Monro, J.D. Adamson, A. Primrose, J.S. McEachern, C.J. Veniot, J.G. Meakins, F.N.G. Starr, L.J. Austin, G.S. Cameron, L. Gérin-Lajoie, G.S. Young, A.G. Nicholls, the author, J.G. Fitzgerald, A.G. Fleming.

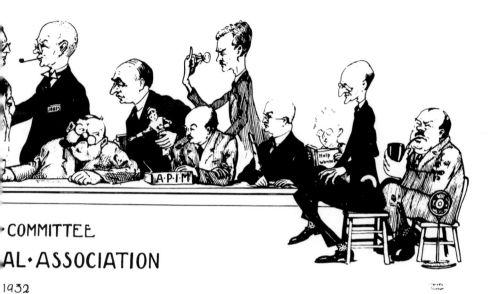

COMMITTEE

AL·ASSOCIATION

1932

OVERLEAF:

The author's portraits of some of his colleagues. Top row: Col Elizabeth Smellie, Percy Ward, T.C. Routley, M.T. MacEachern; bottom: L.O. Bradley, Rev Herbert Wright.

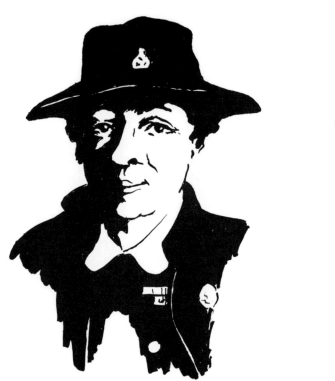
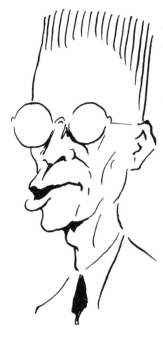
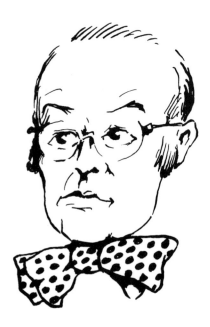

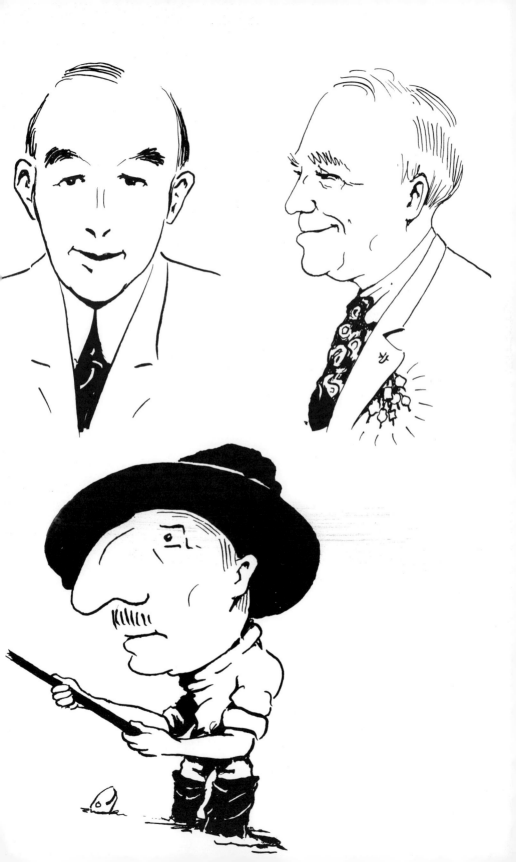

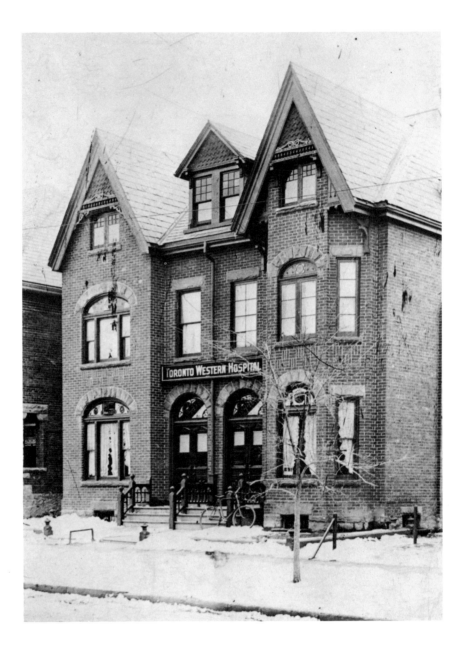

The home in 1895 of the Toronto Western Hospital was this pair of semi-detached houses on Manning Avenue. The building still stands and is used today as a rooming house.

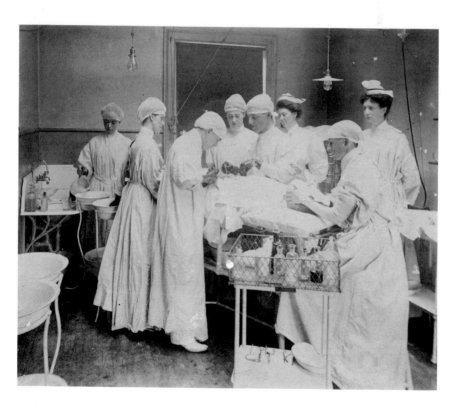

In the light of two shadeless bulbs, a Toronto Western surgical team operates in a
room possibly located in the Manning Avenue building. The photograph is
undated but was taken before the use of masks became obligatory.

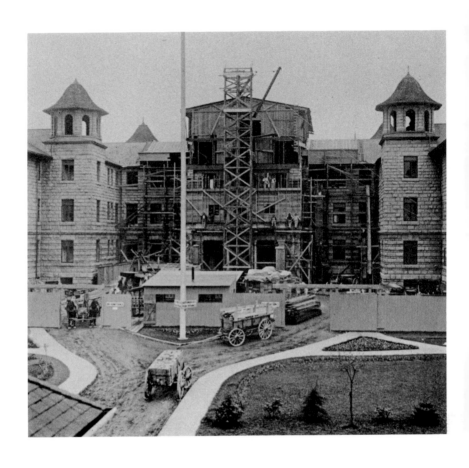

Horse-drawn construction carts line up in front of the Vancouver General Hospital during construction in 1915 of the Heather Pavilion.

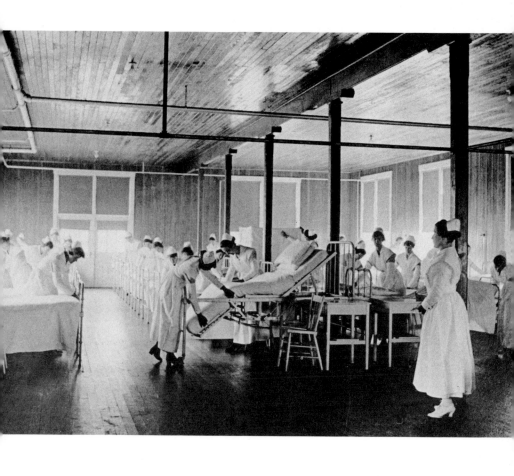

Under the watchful eye of an instructor, student nurses practise bed-making in
the Heather Pavilion after the influenza epidemic of 1918.

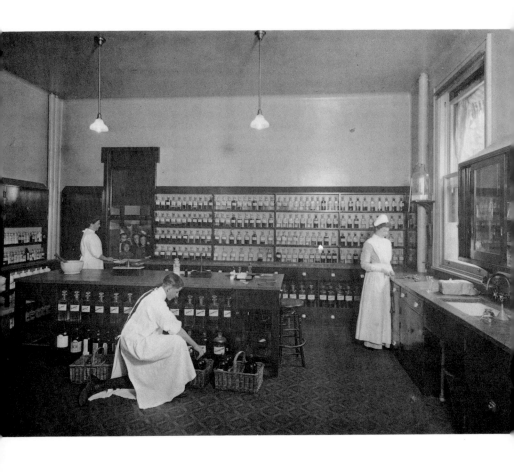

Youngsters on a tour of the Hospital for Sick Children, Toronto, peer through the door of the hospital's dispensary, 1915.

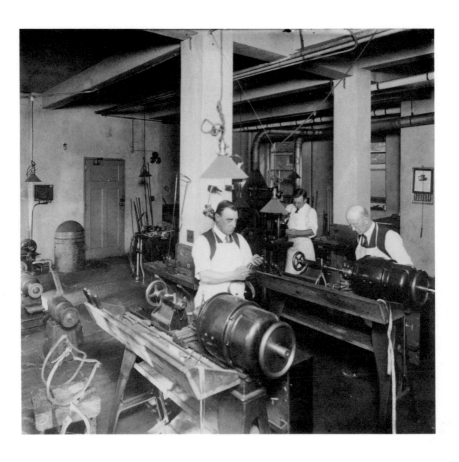

Craftsmen in the same hospital's orthopaedic shop manufacture prosthetics for the patients about 1918.

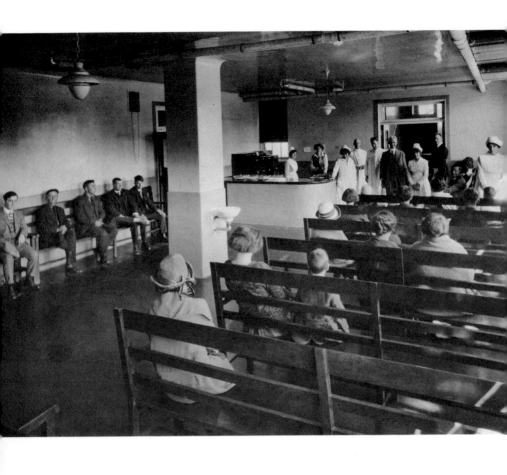

By 1924 the Toronto Western Hospital had moved into a new building on Bathurst Street. This was the outpatient department, with its nursing and medical staff posed with their patients.

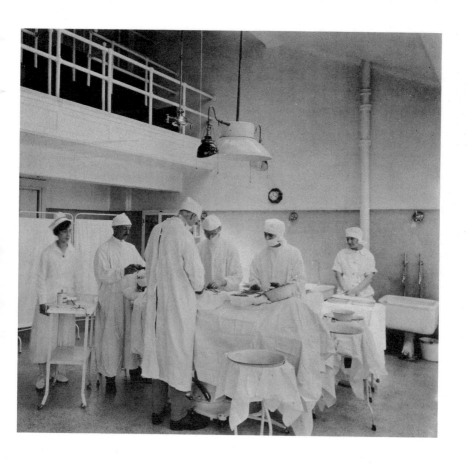

The Toronto Western's south operating room in 1924. The surgeon operated in a gown which covered his street clothes. The gallery was for medical students to observe from.

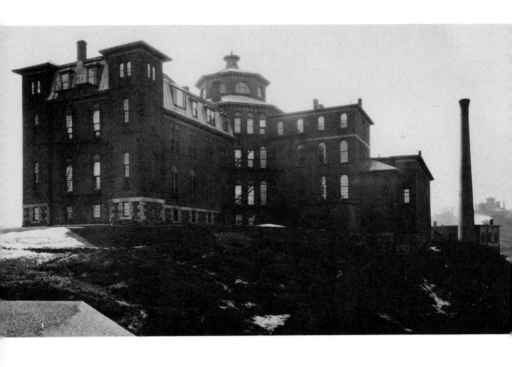

The Saint John, New Brunswick, General Hospital at its completion in 1930.

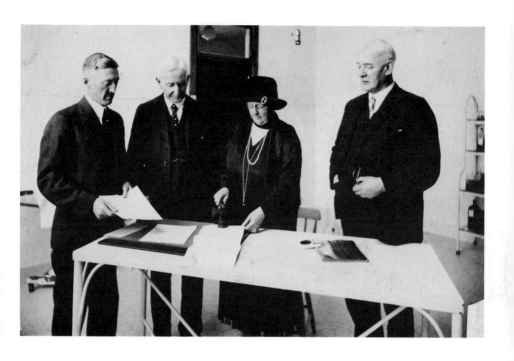

Four members of the board of the Saint John Hospital, officiating at the building's opening.

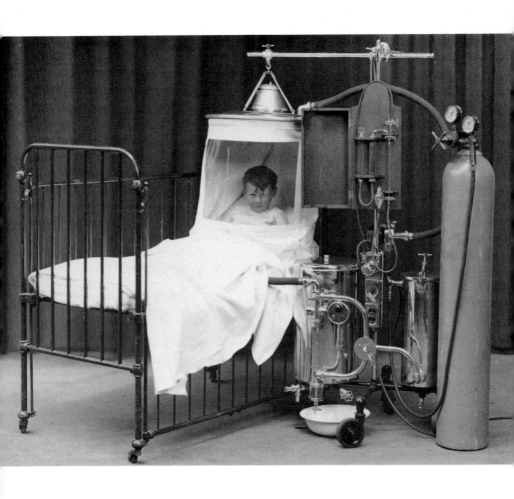

This apparatus was used to supply oxygen to patients in 1930, at the Hospital for Sick Children, Toronto.

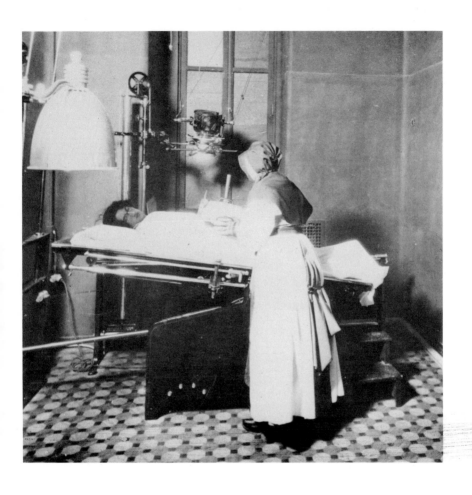

A Sister of Charity from the Grey Nuns of Montreal operates the X-ray machine in the Regina Grey Nuns' Hospital, about 1930.

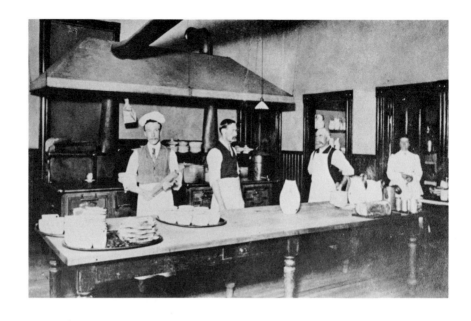

Food services in the Vancouver General Hospital in 1904.

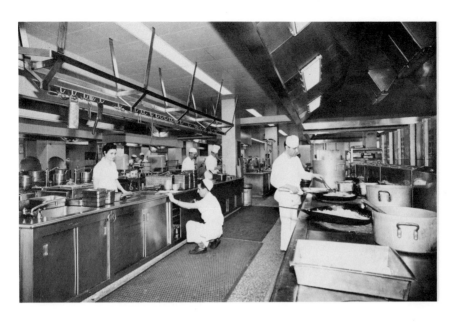

The kitchen of a modern hospital – the Toronto General in 1963.

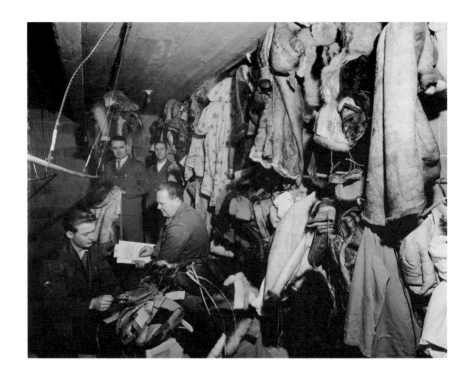

Hospital personnel catalogue and store the fur garments of Eskimo patients at the Charles Camsell Hospital in Edmonton in 1955. The Camsell is operated by the federal Department of Indian Affairs and Northern Development.

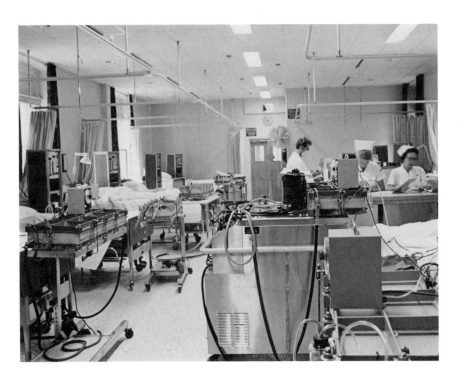

The renal dialysis unit at Vancouver General Hospital in 1969. At the foot of
each bed stand the so-called 'artificial kidneys.'

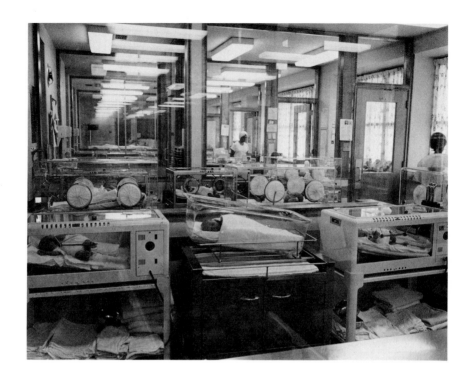

The nursery at Misericordia General Hospital, Winnipeg, as seen in the 1960s through the visitors' window.

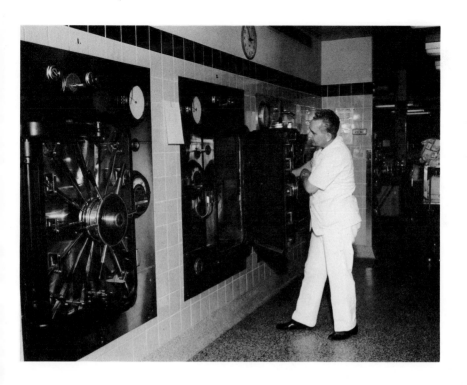

An employee checks the autoclaves in the central sterile supply department of Misericordia General Hospital, Winnipeg, during the mid-sixties.

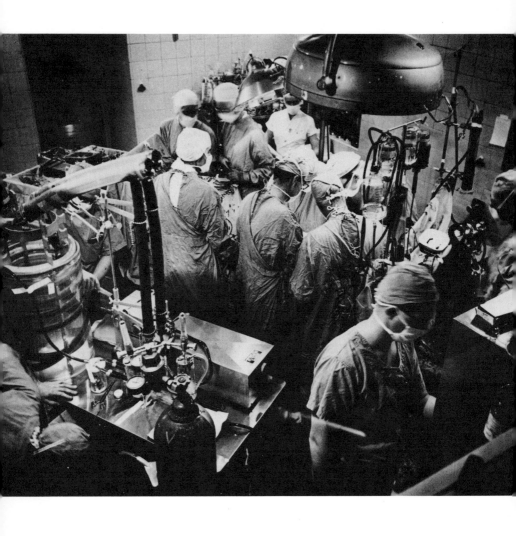

One of the first open-heart surgery teams in Canada was assembled at the Vancouver General Hospital. This photograph shows the team at an operation in 1960.

5

The evolution of hospital financing

During the early decades of the period 1920 to 1970 hospitals struggled constantly to remain solvent. This struggle was greater, naturally, in the voluntary hospital. But even among the municipally owned institutions the reluctance of many municipalities to provide adequate funds made financing a continuing nightmare that haunted trustees and administrators.

Provincial and municipal assistance were minimal for many years. Most provinces paid a per diem grant to voluntary hospitals similar to assistance given orphanages and other charitable institutions. This grant ranged from thirty cents to one dollar and more; but generally it averaged fifty cents per patient per day.[1] This rarely covered more than 20 to 30 percent of the hospital's non-capital costs. In two provinces, New Brunswick and Prince Edward Island, a lump sum was paid to each hospital proportionate to the deficit incurred by the end of the year.

Following the stock market crash in the autumn of 1929, unemployment was everywhere, cash was a curiosity, and credit was just about as scarce. The hospitals suffered the repercussions as much as others. On the Prairies, with the up-and-down fluctuation of crops, many hospitals were already in bad financial shape. Private patients became public ward patients; many of those who remained 'private' didn't pay anyway – they couldn't. Municipalities couldn't pay for their indigents, because taxes couldn't be collected.

---

1 In some cases this grant was applied at first only to indigents (the majority of hospital patients before 1900) but was later expanded to include all patients.

One example will illustrate the experience of many hospitals. S.H. Curran of Yorkton, Saskatchewan, a former president of the Saskatchewan Hospital Association and a tough, practical businessman became chairman of the finance committee of the hospital at Yorkton. Writing from retirement in Vancouver, he recalls how the hospital went 'broke.' He faced a tough job – the hospital owed the bank $30,000; it owed its suppliers about $16,000; it had 'one dime in the bank' and a drawerful of worthless acounts receivable. Under Curran's chairmanship the committee did a lot of trading. It accepted cord wood from rural municipalities for accounts owing and also beef for rural accounts – from individual farmers or from rural municipalities which had taken it in lieu of taxes. Curran traded these goods to the city to give to citizens on relief and he applied the payment on the account with the city.

'I regarded the Hospital as a business concern,' he writes, 'not as a charitable institution, as the charity was all on the part of the Hospital in foregoing payment from patients. But the Hospital did not receive any charity – it had to pay for everything.' Now that it is all over, he adds, 'It really was a lot of fun doing a bit of horse trading,' and he considers the time spent on the hospital 'the most interesting I ever spent – I felt I was doing a bit of good for the community.' The hospital cleared off its debts, too.

In the fine history of the Calgary General Hospital compiled by H. Sadler and his committee in 1955, reference is made to the difficult depression years: 'Relief recipients flocked to the pharmacy where they were issued free drugs. General Hospital graduates, unable to get positions as special nurses, were glad to be taken on the hospital staff at a monthly salary of thirty dollars in addition to room and board. Many supervisory nurses, already on staff, had to take substantial salary reductions as the city slashed and re-slashed its hospital budget in a desperate attempt to make ends meet with the reduced taxes it was able to collect.'

Had the hospital been privately supported rather than municipal it could not have done even that much. I recall many instances where graduate nurses were glad to go on staff for fifteen dollars a month and maintenance. As this history of the Calgary hospital points out, the hospital was flooded with applications from girls wanting go into training; their parents grasped at the chance for free board and room (along with the training, of course). As an aid in selection, the hospital raised its educational requirements to Grade 11. (The sole bright spot of the depression years was the replacement in 1934 of the old high-top boots worn by the nurses, by black oxfords; in 1936, short-sleeved uniforms replaced those long sleeves and stiff white cuffs.)

The doctors faced their own set of difficulties. An increasing proportion of their patients could not pay their bills. Many of the sick called the doctor anyway; others, through consideration for the doctor and sometimes because of personal embarassment, put off medical attention. This often meant a worsening of the condition and, in the long run, an increased amount of medical care. In rural areas barter developed, but there is a limit to the amount of turnips or chickens that a doctor and his family can eat. And of what use is unprocessed rye and barley to a medical man?

Fortunately, a number of provinces extended their welfare provisions; this arrangement helped to meet many of the financial aspects of medical care, although there was a thick stratum of citizens who did not qualify for relief, yet had no cash. It was in this atmosphere that the Social Credit theory of keeping money in constant circulation got wide support, and the low denomination bills with their many stamps affixed were common currency in Alberta.

During the thirties I recall a study completed in British Columbia, a province somewhat better off than other parts of the country during the depression, which demonstrated that only about 40 to 50 percent of the patient days in public hospitals were paid for in full by some 55 to 60 percent of the total number of patients. Another 8 percent of the patients, consuming 10 to 11 percent of the total days care paid part (usually about half) of their hospital bill. About a third of the remaining patients who could not pay were not classified as indigents for grant purposes even though they were often on relief. Monies owing for the services to these patients and others had to be largely written off as bad debts.

In most parts of the country municipalities bore the brunt of the medical and hospital costs of indigents in accordance with the traditions of the Elizabethan Poor Law, and most provinces made provision for the indigent residents of areas not organized municipally. In some cases municipalities contributed extensively and generously to hospital costs. But, generally, both local and provincial authorities were as tight-fisted with their hospital grants as they were with every aspect of their budgets.

In Quebec, hospitals were supported according to the number of indigents accommodated. The province and municipality paid equal grants which totalled less than the proportion of per diem costs they were purported to cover.

In Nova Scotia municipalities paid a set amount (about $2 by the late 1930s) per day toward the cost of each indigent patient. The provincial government paid a per diem grant of thirty cents for many years.

In Ontario municipalities were required to pay a minimum of $1.50 per indigent patient day in 1920. The province paid a per diem grant of fifty cents during the twenties, which was increased to sixty cents in 1928.

In the Prairies the provincial governments made per diem grants of about fifty cents throughout the twenties and thirties. In many areas the hospitals were built and operated through local tax revenues. The development of small, municipally owned hospitals on the Prairies was a logical solution to the problem of providing local hospital accommodation. There was no 'big-house-on-the-hill' to be donated by the family of the former 'lumber king' of the area. In fact the large-scale grain grower (large by eastern standards) could be a wealthy man one year and be living on credit the next year or two. Except for the Sisters' hospitals in larger cities and a few mission hospitals operated by religious groups, there was little place on the Prairies for the voluntary hospital. At this time western Canada did not have the voluntary hospital so popular in the east and in British Columbia. In order to secure the community co-operation required to construct and run a hospital it was often necessary to work through the local municipal government.

Then came the 'union' hospitals where two or more municipalities – usually rural – united to build and support a better hospital than one village or town could do on its own. As early as 1916 in Saskatchwan and 1919 in Alberta legislation was passed authorizing the creation of municipal districts. At first the 'union districts' were formed to combine resources to lure qualified doctors. Subsequently, they were authorized to build and operate hospitals. By 1920 there were ten municipal (or union) hospital areas in Saskatchewan and three in Alberta. The hospital district councils were originally authorized to pay for hospitalization of indigent patients only. Before long, however, hospital care for all the residents of a municipal district was sponsored from the local property taxes.

This was a type of hospital insurance and before municipalities could enter such an arrangement they had to win the support of the local electorate in a referendum. By 1940 municipalities were authorized to levy a poll tax in addition to or instead of the land tax in order to raise hospital funds.

In British Columbia, the provincial government paid $1.25 per diem for the first 1000 patient-days and lesser amounts for the days in excess of that number. Municipal grants were generally not as generous as in other provinces except during the depression when alarming deficits were incurred by hospitals serving large numbers of non-paying transients seeking a milder climate as well as job opportunities in British Columbia.

Some provinces provided financial support to hospitals by subsidizing the costs of various conditions and diseases. Maternity beds were financed at $3 per day in Quebec from the 1930s and comprehensive maternity benefits were provided in Alberta in 1944. By that time free diagnosis and hospitalization were provided for all cancer patients in Alberta and Saskatchewan. Provincial support for institutions providing care for tuberculous and psychiatric patients was well established.

In Ontario, beginning in 1914, the financial burden of industrial accidents and diseases was alleviated through compulsory insurance programs in specific industries. Workmen's compensation was provided for all accidents arising out of and during the course of employment in these industries. Rates were assessed according to the risks of each particular industry or occupation and premiums deducted at source. The injured worker was entitled to comprehensive medical and hospitalization benefits on a semi-private basis (to permit the patient to retain the exclusive attendance of his personal physician). This included all necessary extras except operating room and X-ray expenses. Following Ontario's lead, the provinces introduced workmen's compensation in the following order: Nova Scotia, 1915; British Columbia, 1916; Manitoba, 1916 (liability insurance, followed by full compensation in 1920); Alberta and New Brunswick, 1918; Saskatchewan, 1929; Quebec, 1931; Prince Edward Island, 1949; Newfoundland, 1951.

Federal assistance was usually not available at all (except where a hospital gave service to war veterans or, rather sparingly, for the care of reserve Indians). Maritime hospitals shared in a tonnage fund set up by the federal government to help underwrite the care of ill or injured sailors.

Aside from this limited government assistance the hospitals were very much on their own.

A fairly sharp division was usually drawn between paying and non-paying patients. Patients in private rooms paid $5 or $6 per day. Semi-public rates were a little lower, and partially because many of the patients in this category were sponsored by the workmen's compensation boards, care was provided at the average per diem cost for the hospital. Paying public ward patients during the twenties usually paid $1.25 to $1.75 per day.[2] Operating room charges were usually $8 to $10, and less for minor surgery.

---

2 Some hospitals received assistance from district or county authorities as well as the municipality and province, and as a result charged a variety of rates for public ward depending on the domicile of the patient. A good example is the Brantford County Hospital in Ontario which throughout the 1920s and 1930s charged seventy cents per day for patients resident in the City of Brantford, $1.50 for patients living outside the city but in Brant County, and $1.75 for patients living outside the county. The reason was that the city subsidized the hospital care of its residents by $1.05 per patient day and the county gave twenty-five cents. Outsiders whose care was likely to be subsidized only by the province had to pay the highest rate.

This charge included anaesthetic material but not medical fees. Out-patient department services (where not delivered free to the patient), varied from a basic charge of ten to fifty cents. Medicines and special items were often charged as extras.

Medical services were free to indigents on the public wards. In the teaching hospitals they were usually free to all public ward patients. In most urban, non-teaching hospitals and in practically all rural or small centre hospitals, non-indigent public ward patients were still considered private and paid a fee, sometimes reduced, to the doctor in charge. Medical services in the emergency or out-patient departments were usually donated by the doctors, although, in some larger hospitals with heavy out-patient or emergency loads, an honorarium was paid to some of the doctors devoting a great deal of time to these services.

The private room charge, as previously implied, was usually a little higher than the average per diem cost. If the average per diem cost amounted to $3 to $3.50, the private room charge would likely be $4.50 to $5.50. The semi-private charge was not far off the average cost per patient-day and the public ward charge was well below cost. The hospital made up a little of its deficit by its private room income and through extras such as the operating room or delivery room fee.

Hospitals operated by Sisters also got some benefits – or the order did – by the donation of the nuns' services. For many years direct charges for the Sisters' services were not computed but, later, when Blue Cross and other payments to hospitals became related to the actual cost of operation, a dollar valuation was placed upon these services. At first the amounts were nominal but later they were equated to what was being paid in other hospitals for comparable services.

The major concern of the hospitals was to get some return for the care of indigents. It was not easy in most instances to determine indigency. Municipal clerks were past masters in retaining the citizens' tax money and the patient and his relatives had to be flat broke to qualify. A small equity in a decrepit cottage or in a worn-out farm meant rejection or the hanging of a collectable debt over the patient's head for his lifetime. Registration on relief rolls was not justification enough to be considered indigent. It took many years for it to be generally recognized that an individual could be 'medically indigent' yet earning money – although barely enough to support a family, usually a large one.

Also it was often very difficult to establish residency in a community. Naturally a municipality had to protect itself from the claims of transients. All provinces had definitions of what constituted residency. In some cases it was unbroken residency for a period of months – at least three and in one instance at least twelve. In Ontario residency was defined as presence in the province during three of the previous twelve months. With some occupational groups like tobacco workers or lumberjacks, the formula for residency could not be met and no municipal payment could be obtained. Administrators and selected trustees were constantly in attendance at county council meetings soliciting payment.

Unless a hospital was one of the few with adequate endowments, it usually had a deficit at the end of the fiscal year. In some hospitals with a large patient and out-patient non-paying clientele (such as children's hospitals or downtown urban hospitals) the deficit was often of alarming proportion.

Some voluntary hospitals received substantial monetary assistance from well-to-do members of their boards. But most voluntary hospitals were not so fortunate and could only clear their extensive overdraft by strenuous effort. Often this required a local campaign to raise funds, an enterprise never so well received as one for new buildings. Sometimes the local hospitals joined together in a common campaign. Frequently the local municipalities, or (less often) provincial authorities, were appealed to and contributed tax funds toward the deficit. It was a recurring situation for the majority of voluntary hospitals and also one of concern to the municipal hospitals.

Some municipal hospital districts on the Prairies restricted the types of service they would sponsor during the financial pinch of the thirties. One example occurred in Yorkton where the municipality would guarantee payment only for emergencies in which life – not just health – was endangered.

It was in the continuous atmosphere of experiences like these that hospital administrators, municipal officials and the public generally began to look for better solutions to hospital payments.

HOSPITAL AND MEDICAL INSURANCE – VOLUNTARY PLANS

The inclination of many in the health field was to turn to the principles of insurance, not only to alleviate the hospitals' problems in collecting accounts but primarily to remove the difficulties and hardships faced by many patients in meeting growing health care costs.

Several small prepayment plans for hospital care had existed for quite a few years across Canada, mainly in the industrial and mining areas of Cape Breton and in connection with some of the smaller hospitals of British Columbia where some of the co-operative principles developed in Great Britain had been applied to prepayment plans. By 1934 a survey conducted by a committee of the Canadian Medical Association documented some twenty-five prepayment plans organized by hospitals, as well as others in which indemnities were provided by sponsoring service clubs, mutual benefit societies, and similar organizations. Medical and hospital insurance was not provided by commercial insurance companies in Canada until the mid-1930s.

The typical policy paid an indemnity of $5 per day in hospital up to a maximum of twenty-one days. The life insurance and casualty insurance companies entering the field were reasonably competitive and a great variety of plans, including some which offered highly comprehensive benefits for hospital care, were introduced during the 1940s and 1950s.

Generally the benefits included in the hospital-run plans were standard ward care and varying degrees of medical attendance and services. Premiums were usually about fifty cents per month. Often initiated and operated in co-operation with local industries (such as the mining interests in Glace Bay, Nova Scotia, Timmins, Ontario, and Trail, British Columbia), enrolment was often restricted to employees of the industry and their dependents.

Although these plans contained the germ of the concept that ultimately broadened into plans with millions of members, this potential had never been explored fully. The impetus came in the early thirties with the success of the teachers' hospitalization plan at Baylor University in Texas.

Bryce Twitty, an indefatigable hospital administrator from Texas, told and re-told the story of the Baylor University plan at American Hospital Association conventions across the continent. He brought along with him key personnel in the plan's administration to answer questions. Because of these discussions various states and provinces became interested, interest that ultimately culminated in the Blue Cross movement.

The Edmonton Group Hospitalization Plan
When Dr A.F. Anderson of the Royal Alexandra Hospital in Edmonton and Dr R.T. Washburn of the University Hospital returned from the 1933 AHA convention, they said to each other, 'Well, what are we waiting for?' Characteristically, they didn't waste any time. The depression still held most persons in a grip of defeatism. Not Anderson and Washburn. They launched the Edmonton Group Hospitalization Plan, with the four Edmonton general hospitals – the Misericordia, the Edmonton General, the University Hospital and the Royal Alexandra – as sponsors. The hospitals constituted themselves a co-operative group and offered stated hospitalization benefits for certain prepaid fees. It was an effort not without risk for

the hospitals to work out the multitude of details of the contracts. They took on the task without flinching.

Initial officers were: General Hospital, Milton Martin; Misericordia, Joseph Pilon; University Hospital, Dr R.T. Washburn; Royal Alexandra, Dr A.F. Anderson. Joseph Monaghan was appointed chief executive officer.

An Albertan to the core, 'Andy' Anderson, one of the driving forces behind the Edmonton plan, was, for many years, a colorful figure at hospital meetings. He took most of his medical course at the old Trinity Medical School in Toronto, went west on one of the then popular harvester excursions, didn't have enough money to get back and so finished his course at the University of Manitoba. After practising for a while in Manitoba, he went to Edmonton where he established a reputation in internal medicine and taught on the staff of the Faculty of Medicine in the University of Alberta during the 1920s. He was medical superintendent of the Royal Alexandra Hospital from 1928 to 1949, succeeding Dr H.R. Smith and being succeeded by Dr Don R. Easton. He ruled with an iron hand guided by plenty of horse sense.

Andy could always be counted on to liven up a business session of his association. Sooner or later something would come up that infringed, or could be construed as likely to infringe, upon hospitals in general, or upon Alberta hospitals as a whole, or upon municipal hospitals as a class (the Royal 'Alex' was city-owned) or upon his own hospital in particular. Andy never failed to let them have it – both barrels at once. Any provincial minister at the meeting knew exactly where the hospitals stood, for, except on rare occasions, where Andy stood so stood the hospitals. A visiting speaker once remarked that he spoke of certain government officials, derelict in their consideration of the hospitals, with the same tonal inflections used by Sir Winston Churchill when he spoke of the Nazis.

As the years passed and the broad shoulders began to droop a little and a cane became helpful, Andy got to his feet more slowly and he took longer to warm up. But the old fire was still there, the wide open light blue eyes still flashed and his points were now accentuated by a vehement pounding of the floor with his sturdy cane. Two interests brightened and lengthened his period of retirement – his love of curling and his pride in his son, Walter, who was surgeon-in-chief at the Royal Alex for many years, and retired as chief in 1971.

The Edmonton plan has been considered to be the first Blue Cross development in Canada. It met with such success that its extension to the province as a whole was inevitable.

By 1948, the Alberta Hospital Association, with the co-operation of the Edmonton group, decided to sponsor and operate a province-wide Blue Cross program. The Edmonton program, after almost fifteen years of operation, provided the necessary experience and a substantial nucleus of policy holders. Dr Angus C. McGugan was the first president of the Alberta Blue Cross Plan and Joseph Monaghan continued his energetic services as executive director. Enrolment expanded for the next ten years to 158,000 subscribers in 1958. In 1971 the supplemental hospital insurance covered almost one million participants.

Angus McGugan, the first president of Alberta Blue Cross, is a member of that little coterie of dedicated Albertans whose great delight as avocational historians has been to record for posterity the achievements of those pioneers who laid such a fine foundation for the health program of this province. We link him with Dr Herbert C. Jamieson, who wrote *Early Medicine in Alberta*; Dr C.D. Stanley, who edited the famous *Historical Bulletin* of the Calgary Associate Clinic; and Dr Earle P. Scarlett, who has long been recognized as having the most erudite pen among Canadian physicians.

Armed with an MD from Alberta (1929) and, later, DPH from Toronto, Dr McGugan joined the Department of Health in Alberta, in turn directing the fight against communicable disease, then serving as medical officer of the Provincial Mental Hospital at Ponoka, then as medical inspector of hospitals and assistant deputy minister of health for the province from 1938 to 1942. For seventeen years thereafter he was superintendent of the University of Alberta Hospital in Edmonton. As noted above he was president for a term of the Associated Hospitals of Alberta, was a valued member of the Canadian Hospital Council (Association) executive for ten years and its president from 1953 to 1955. He was general co-ordinator of the Western Canada Institute for nine years, was a fellow and regent (Western Canada) of the American College of Hospital Administrators, was chairman of the first board of trustees of the Alberta Blue Cross Plan and a member of the House of Delegates of the American Hospital Association. In 1959 he received the George Findlay Stephens Memorial Award for outstanding service. In the sixties he found time to serve his fellow citizens as an alderman.

Dr McGugan's career illustrates the old adage that, if you want something done, give it to a busy man.

Manitoba Blue Cross and other provincial plans
In 1937, largely due to the efforts of Dr George Stephens of the Winnipeg General, W.T. Hunt, Dr O.C. Trainor, Dr E.C. Moorhead and many

others, the Manitoba Hospital Service Association was created by a special act of the Manitoba legislature to administer a province-wide Blue Cross Plan. Under the sponsorship of the Winnipeg Council of Social Agencies, intense studies of plans operating in the United States were conducted in 1937 and 1938. The provincial hospital and medical associations were guaranteed representation (not a majority) on the board of trustees of the new MHSA, the remaining members to be appointed by voluntary and government agencies. The plan went into full-scale operation in January 1939 and was the first *official* Blue Cross plan in Canada.

Other provinces rapidly followed suit: Ontario in 1941, Quebec in 1942, the Maritimes and British Columbia in 1943. In 1949 Newfoundland citizens became eligible for coverage under the Maritime program, although fairly comprehensive health insurance had in fact been available to many Newfoundlanders since 1935 under the Cottage Hospital and Medical Care Plan.

The Quebec Blue Cross plan, operated under the name of the Quebec Hospital Service Association, was similar in its organization to the Manitoba plan – it was administered by a combination of hospitals and medical association representatives, as well as representatives of charitable institutions, business, labor and education. Dr George Stephens, who had moved from Winnipeg to Montreal in 1940, was eager to help organize the Blue Cross Insurance Plan in Quebec following his successful experience in Manitoba. He found a great deal of enthusiasm for Blue Cross in Montreal not only in the hospital field but in organized medicine and throughout sectors of society. J.R.H. Robertson, H.C. Hayes, G.C. McDonald, and Edgar Genest were some of the members of the executive committee in the early years. Besides Dr Stephens, J.H. Roy, Dr A.L.C. Gilday, S.S. Cohen, Réné Laporte and Dr Eugene Thibault were representatives of the Montreal Hospital Council. Duncan Millican was the director of the plan.

Joseph Roy, one of the original members of the Montreal council, long director of l'Hôpital St Luc in Montreal, was the council president for twenty-one years and a key supporter of the fledgling Canadian Hospital Council in the thirties; he helped to organize the Quebec Hospital Service Association (Blue Cross) in 1942; was a Fellow of the ACHA; and richly deserved the George Findlay Stephens Award in 1958. It may be because of his great dedication, but did anyone ever see Joe smile?

As the plan expanded throughout the province, representation was extended to advisory committees from Quebec City and the Eastern Townships. Representation was also extended to le Comité des Hôpitaux as that group became consolidated in the early fifties, and to medical societies representing doctors across the province after supplemental medical insurance was introduced by the OHSA in 1948.

The Maritime Hospital Service Association, which ran Blue Cross in the Maritimes, was wholly sponsored by the Maritime Hospital Association and members of the board of directors were appointed on a geographic basis for many years. Only when medical and surgical insurance was provided in addition to the basic hospital plan was it considered necessary to extend board representation to the medical profession and the subscribers.

Dr J.A. McMillan and Ruth Wilson were the first president and executive director respectively of the Blue Cross Plan in the Maritimes.

In Alberta and Ontario the Blue Cross Plans were organized as direct subsidiaries of the hospital associations in each province.

In the case of Alberta, a separate board of directors was organized, but it was appointed by the parent board of the hospital association.

In Ontario the Blue Cross Plan was administered by a committee of the OHA composed, like other OHA committees, of hospital trustees and administrators. The rapid growth of the plan during the forties and fifties necessitated the employment of hundreds of full-time staff. Health insurance became the most ambitious undertaking of the association.

The insurance plans as such were markedly similar in their methods of operations and benefits offered. They were all non-profit, voluntary, provided service benefits in terms of hospital care and required prepayment from subscribers. Cautious at first, they usually started by offering only one or two standard contracts designed to build up an adequate reserve fund (totalling three months of hospital benefits and operating expenses) required by the Blue Cross Commission of the American Hospital Association. Benefits usually included up to twenty-one days of hospital bed and board, general nursing service, operating room services, anaesthetics, lab services, ordinary drugs, dressing, casts, electrocardiographic films and basal metabolism tests. Maternity benefits were provided after a subscriber or his dependents had been enrolled for ten to twelve months. Generally not included were serums, vaccines, expensive drugs, oxygen therapy, ambulatory service, private nurses, and, of course, the services of private physicians.

Originally enrolment was restricted to employee groups, or in some cases professional groups, of five persons or more. Standard ward care and semi-private care plans were offered. For standard ward care premiums were fifty cents per month for a single subscriber and one dollar per month for a family. Semi-private care rates were seventy-five cents and $1.50 (at least until 1945). As the plans became established and financially secure the scope of benefits was enlarged. Premiums were raised to provide for the increased benefits and for the rising costs of hospital services.

In the late forties and early fifties some of the Blue Cross organizations added supplemental medical and surgical insurance to the basic hospital coverage. The benefits offered were indemnities as it proved impractical to get the majority of doctors to participate in providing service benefits on a provincial scope without control of the plan by the doctors themselves. There was, of course, little difficulty in getting hospitals to agree to accept Blue Cross payments, not only because it helped alleviate the hospitals' financial problems but also because in most provinces operating Blue Cross provincial hospital association membership was contingent upon participation in the plan.

In any case, the Blue Cross plans were all devoted to the ultimate ideal of totally comprehensive hospital insurance. In fact, in Quebec, the Hospital Service Association made efforts in the late fifties to extend its coverage to include welfare benefits through the sponsorship of the Quebec Mutual Life Assurance Company.

Enrolment grew very quickly in most parts of the country with the notable exception of British Columbia. In that province the Blue Cross Plan managed to enrol well over one hundred thousand participants in its five years of operation but this represented less than 15 percent of the British Columbian population. In other provinces, however, the plans had to make herculean efforts to meet the demand for enrolment. In Manitoba, participation increased from some 22,000 subscribers and dependents in December 1939 to more than 56,000 in 1941. This had increased to almost 187,000 participants by the end of 1945, 289,000 by 1950, and in 1958 when compulsory government-sponsored hospital insurance went into effect in Manitoba some 415,000 persons or about 45 per cent of the population were covered by Blue Cross. In Ontario approximately 2,250,000 people were enrolled in Blue Cross in 1958.

Upon the introduction of government-sponsored hospitalization in the late 1950s, only Manitoba Blue Cross decided to cease operations. The others revamped their coverage to include only those benefits not covered by the government plans. Ontario, the Maritimes, Quebec and Alberta have had considerable success in operating prepayment insurance plans for semi-private care, extended health care, prescription drugs, dental care and other benefits. The Quebec and Maritimes plans continue to offer medical benefits (indemnities) supplemental to the basic government insurance. In Ontario some 3.5 million subscribers were covered by Blue Cross in

1970. In Quebec, Blue Cross enrolment was more than one million in the same year.

Fortunately the Blue Cross plans in Canada and the hospitals have not had the serious clashes which have occurred in recent years in the United States. There, much disagreement has arisen respecting payments and various hospital groups have dissociated themselves from the regional Blue Cross plan, usually on the basis of the inadequacy of payment for the care of Blue Cross patients. The happier Canadian situation has been due, in part, to the close association of the Blue Cross plans with the hospitals, either by actual integration with their associations or through the individuals directing them or on their boards. Another factor has been that, in this country, provincially sponsored hospital insurance plans came into being early in this present period of escalating costs, increasing unionization, and rising deficits. With operating budgets adjusted annually, hospitals here, despite varying restrictions, are not in such desperate financial straits as are some of their American counterparts.

MEDICAL INSURANCE

Although technically not part of the hospital bill, the fees of personal physicians sometimes presented an additional financial hardship for the hospital patient. Most physicians were acutely aware of the obstacles which high medical costs, especially those accumulated on top of a substantial hospital bill, often presented to the delivery of good health care, and to good doctor-patient relationships. In the twenties and thirties medical fees composed a much higher proportion of total health costs. For these reasons and others a proliferation of voluntary medical insurance plans sprang up in the late thirties and forties. They began in 1937 with Dr J.A. Hannah's Associated Medical Services based in Toronto and endorsed by the Ontario Medical Association and the Civil Service Association of Ontario. This was the first of nine plans sponsored by the medical associations which offered generally comprehensive service benefits including office and home calls. Others included the Windsor Medical Society Plan, 1939; Regina Medical Services, 1939; Medical Services Associated of British Columbia, 1940; Manitoba Medical Services, 1942; Medical Services Incorporated, Saskatoon, 1946; Physicians Services Incorporated, Ontario, 1947; Medical Services Incorporated, Alberta, 1948; Maritime Medical Care Incorporated, Nova Scotia, 1948.

The Swift Current (Saskatchewan) Plan, although not sponsored and controlled by a medical association, offered equally comprehensive benefits. All medical fees incurred for hospital care were covered up to a prescribed schedule except for services covered by hospital insurance plans. (This usually occurred where the anaesthetist or other specialist was on the payroll of the hospital.)

During the fifties the Canadian Medical Association attempted to establish a co-ordinating mechanism for the various doctor-sponsored plans. Trans-Canada Medical Services was set up to attempt to standardize the coverage and operation of the individual plans. Enrolment in medical insurance plans, while not so extensive as in the Blue Cross plans, almost quadrupled during the 1950s to more than four million.

During the sixties compulsory government-sponsored medical insurance became universal. Beginning in Saskatchewan in 1961, events moved rapidly and culminated in the federal Medical Care Act of 1968.

For some years the medical profession exhibited mixed sentiments respecting health insurance. Many doctors believed there were great dangers of third-party interference with the close relationship of patient and physician. Others swore they would only work on a fee-for-service basis and were wary of having to limit their practice to one geographic area. Others feared having to take orders regarding medical treatment from a bureaucratic organization, perhaps under non-medical direction. Still others feared lower incomes and political promotions. Certain obvious failures of the British system of medical insurance were cited endlessly as inevitable faults of *any* health insurance scheme.

As secretary of the committee on economics of the Canadian Medical Association for many years, I saw and heard these concerns, and I have been convinced over the years that the greatest factor in making the medical profession ultra-conservative in viewpoint is fear of the unknown. Many doctors saw health insurance rapidly evolving into state medicine and their fears were not assuaged by some radical groups pressing for health insurance with ill-prepared enthusiasm.

In 1934 the CMA recommended that if health insurance were introduced it should be along principles outlined in a model plan. It was not until 1943, however, that the CMA took a stand and asserted that health insurance *should* be introduced. The resolution passed at a special meeting of the council in Ottawa in January of that year stated that:

1 The Canadian Medical Association approves the adoption of the principle of Health Insurance.

2 The Canadian Medical Association favours a plan of Health Insurance which will secure other development and provision of the highest standard of health

services, preventive and curative, if such plan be fair both to the insured and to all those rendering the services.[3]

It is difficult to judge the ultimate importance of this endorsation but one cannot help but reflect on the experience in the United States, where health insurance has been so long delayed in some measure by the stringent opposition of the American Medical Association.

THE GOVERNMENT-SPONSORED INSURANCE PLANS

There are many reasons why the provincial and federal governments have become involved actively in the provision of universal health insurance. Society at large has been concerned for years about gaps between the advances and discoveries of medical science and the means to deliver these benefits to everyone regardless of income. Shortages of professional personnel (especially physicians and nurses), hospitals and modern equipment were all worrisome. But of particular consternation were the difficulties that many people were having in meeting hospital and medical costs. Linked to the personal or familial difficulty in meeting medical costs were the financial problems of the hospitals themselves. These problems and difficulties were considerably aggravated by the depression and the second world war.

Government spending in the health sector has always been limited (to some extent) by other priorities in education, welfare, highway building and other areas. The resources necessary to provide expanding programs in all of these areas simply weren't available to the provinces with their limited tax base. The most satisfactory solution seemed to be the granting of monies by the federal government to the provinces so that the latter could fulfill their obligations adequately.

But the federal government objected to the initiation of any new aid programs during the depression or later during the second world war, and provinces which wanted to establish a health insurance program had to contemplate going it alone.

The western provinces had been interested for some time in subsidized medical and hospital insurance plans. Legislative committees, royal commissions and various other studies had been charged with exploring the possibilities of such programs. For example, the British Columbia government appointed royal commissions in 1919 and 1929, both of which recom-

3 From the minutes of the special meeting.

mended the introduction of government-sponsored health insurance. The first report was discarded after confusion arose over the respective jurisdictions of federal and provincial authorities. The second report, issued in 1932, was eagerly taken up by the Honorable George Weir, provincial secretary in the Patullo cabinet,[4] and a health insurance bill was passed in 1936. The major reason the bill was never promulgated was primarily because the premier, urged on by the provincial treasurer, John Hart, decided that the province could not afford it. The plan was also opposed by the British Columbia Medical Association on the grounds that indigent persons were not covered.

In Alberta a comprehensive health insurance act was similarly passed but never promulgated in 1935. In Saskatchewan and Manitoba considerable interest existed among the legislators and various studies were commissioned.

The provincial governments east of Manitoba took very little interest in provincially sponsored health insurance in the twenties and thirties although in the early forties a Health Insurance Commission was set up in Quebec as a preliminary step to a government insurance program. This commission was disbanded in 1945 after a change in government.

The federal government had little responsibility for legislation concerning health insurance but it was generally sympathetic to demands that it contribute financial aid to provincial programs. The Honorable W.L. Mackenzie King inserted a proposal for health insurance into the platform of the Liberal party in 1919. Furthermore, grants-in-aid had been used effectively in other areas such as highway construction, vocational training, and venereal disease control.

The report of the standing committee on industrial and international relations of the House of Commons in 1929 recommended that 'with regard to sickness insurance, the Department of Pensions and National Health be requested to initiate a comprehensive survey of the field of public health, with special reference to a national health programme.' This report was approved by the Dominion Council of Health in 1933.

In 1935 the Employment and Social Insurance Act, subsequently declared unconstitutional in the courts, established a commission to gather data and serve in an advisory capacity to provincial agencies or groups planning a health insurance program.

---

4 In British Columbia, prior to October 1946, the administration of the Health Act, the Hospital Act and the Hospital Insurance Act was the responsibility of the Department of the Provincial Secretary.

Citing the 1929 report, the federal government set up in February 1942 an advisory committee on health insurance under Dr J.J. Heagerty, federal Director of Public Health Services. Briefs were invited from health, welfare and other interested national organizations. It was at this time that the Canadian Medical Association, which had been debating the issue for a number of years, decided to endorse the principles of health insurance and the formation of 'fair' hospital and medical insurance programs.

While it recommended a fee-for-service basis of payment for medical specialists, the Canadian Medical Association recognized that a capitation or salary basis as well as fee-for-service method might prove desirable in the case of general practioners. The decision was to be left to the individual province in consultation with the doctors to be affected.

Dr Heagerty's committee advocated grants-in-aid to provinces enacting legislation similar to that outlined in a model provincial health insurance bill. In addition grants would be given to provinces instituting preventive health programs which met federal standards. All grants were to be contingent on the introduction of the detailed insurance plan. The report of the advisory committee was submitted to the Honorable Cyrus McMillan's House of Commons special committee on social security in January 1943. Throughout that year and 1944 the committee held weeks of hearings. The provinces were consulted and numerous alterations were made to attempt to meet objections, the foremost of which was that the federal government was eroding provincial jurisdiction by insisting on standards and methods that were rigid and too detailed.

Unfortunately, dominion-provincial conferences following the war became bogged down in disagreements over general revenue sources and distribution. As a result, agreements over grants-in-aid in the health field were delayed for several years.

In the meantime, Saskatchewan under Premier T.C. Douglas was taking steps to set up a hospital insurance plan financed through its own resources. Blue Cross had never existed in that province but, impressed by the performance of such plans elsewhere, the political and medical leaders incorporated many elements of Blue Cross into the new plan. For many years municipal doctor and municipal hospital plans had provided insurance financed through land (later poll) taxes for much of the rural population. In 1946 there were more than one hundred municipal hospital districts in Saskatchewan. The new compulsory plan was adapted to the old system so that the premiums were still collected locally once a year. Registration, too, was decentralized. Because municipal clerks knew virtually everyone residing in the hospital districts, near-universal coverage was achieved much more easily than in British Columbia, where several years later many persons, including lumberjacks and other transients, successfully ignored the compulsory registration.

The Saskatchewan plan was financed by a premium tax of five dollars per capita to a maximum of $30 per family. The provincial government subsidized the plan with funds from general revenues approximately equivalent to previous per diem payments, cancer patient payments and others. In the second year of operation (1948) rising hospital costs made it necessary to increase the sales tax.

The plan originally paid hospitals a per diem grant according to the quality and extent of facilities and services provided in order to create an incentive for better care. Unfortunately the costs of providing a given level of service varied somewhat and some hospitals ran deficits which the government was obliged to cover, thereby negating the incentive. Also, various elaborate facilities were developed where a real need for them did not exist. Funding was directly proportional to occupancy, thereby causing uneven flows of monies and financial hardship during low occupancy. Eventually, payments were made on a fixed-plus-variable cost scheme so that approximately 80 percent of a hospital's estimated required revenues were paid regardless of occupancy. This partially removed financial motives for the hospital to keep its beds full at all times through lax admission and discharge practices.

British Columbia introduced compulsory hospital insurance in 1949. The plan ran into trouble immediately when many avoided premium collections and revenues fell considerably below expectation. Payment through payroll deduction was made compulsory where possible but it was not until the province switched completely to sales tax financing in 1954 that the situation was rectified completely.

In Saskatchewan the plan was administered by a representative commission of five until 1950, at which time the responsibility was transferred to the Department of Public Health and a new purely advisory committee was formed. In British Columbia a single commissioner administered the program and was directly responsible to the minister of health. In 1959 he became the deputy minister of hospital insurance.

In 1949 Alberta introduced a new program of subsidizing the municipal hospital district plans to approximately 50 percent of the costs of standard ward care. Deterrent charges of a dollar per day (or $2 per day if the municipal plan coverage was more extensive) were maintained.

On the federal scene, the Honorable Ian Mackenzie, Dr Heagerty, myself and others held extensive conversations. It soon became apparent that no plan of health insurance providing hospital coverage with little or no immediate cost to the patient could operate without widespread criticism unless a reasonably adequate number of beds were to be available. The current supply of beds was inadequate in most Canadian communities. The increasing complexity of medical diagnosis and treatment, coupled with an ever more noticeable shortage of physicians and nurses, was putting an increasing strain on hospital accommodation. The simple economics of the increasing cost of additions or of modernization was making it more and more difficult for the hospitals to finance these necessary construction programs. A few provinces were beginning to make small capital grants to voluntary hospitals (the first being Saskatchewan in 1944). A much more ambitious program was needed, however.

The Canadian Hospital Council proposed to the federal minister of pensions and national health (national health and welfare from 1945) that low-interest federal loans would be a possible solution. This would not be trespassing on provincial jurisdiction unduly and would be an extension of the principle of federal assistance which could be justified without difficulty.

A few years before, the Beveridge report had come out in Great Britain and Lord Beveridge appeared before the Canadian House of Commons committee. His proposals and recommendations were scrutinized carefully.

Of more immediate impact was the Hill-Burton Act of 1946 in the United States which authorized federal assistance to hospitals so that the latter might keep up with the demand for more accommodation and facilities. Large sums were allotted to the different states, the per capita amount varying with the overall affluence of the state and its ability to help its own hospitals. The stimulus this act provided was tremendous and resulted in an extensive hospital expansion program across the United States.

It was a stimulus in others ways, too. Many of the states had poor hospital enactments and regulations. Some had poor statistical knowledge of their hospital activities. Six or eight – New York, Pennsylvania, Ohio and others – had good state supervision and knowledge of their hospitals. A primary requirement for qualifying for federal assistance was the legislating of adequate state laws and regulations and a state-wide appraisal of the degree of obsolescence of each hospital. Priorities for assistance were established and all grants were processed by a state Hill-Burton committee. This development was being watched in Canada with close interest. Some of us in Canada had been of help to a few of the states and the American Hospital Association concerning legislative detail because of our experience with progressive provincial legislation and hospital-provincial relationships. The Hill-Burton Basis of aid was superior to what we were asking in Canada.

One morning in 1948 the phone in the Canadian Hospital Council office rang and I was told the Honorable C.D. Howe was coming on the line. The cabinet was about to meet and he was going into the meeting with a proposal. At least, that was my conjecture, for he wasted no time on pleasantries or explanation.

'If we give grants to your hospitals instead of low-interest loans, how much do you want?'

'Well, Mr Howe,' I replied, 'We haven't got that far in our thinking; however, I can obtain that figure for you.'

'That won't do,' he snapped, 'I want a figure right now.'

I had to pull a figure out of the air.

'All right,' I said, 'Thirty million a year.'

'Fine,' and he banged down the receiver.

Two or three weeks later we read in the newspaper that the federal government had approved $65 million over five years towards hospital construction. This was to be on a matching basis – $1,000 per active-treatment bed[5] from Ottawa and the same from the province for each new bed or approved replacement; for certain clinical services this $1,000 would apply to each 1,000 square feet of space provided. In 1958 this sum was increased to $2,000 per bed.

The national health grants program consisted, in fact, of four different types of grants. One was to finance a survey of the existing health services and facilities within the province 'to insure the most effective use of the other three health grants and in planning the expansion of hospital accomodation and the proper organization of hospital and medical care insurance.' The others were the hospital construction grants, grants in support of public health, mental health and other existing programs, and grants for professional training.

The construction grants were of tremendous value in increasing available beds and other hospital facilities. In the first five years an additional 46,000 beds were provided and 4,600 new health workers were added to hospital staffs. By the time most provinces had introduced hospital insurance in the late fifties, more than 40,000 acute general hospital beds, almost 20,000 mental hospital beds, more than 7,000 chronic and convalescent care beds and about 4,500 beds in tuberculosis sanatoria had been built – all since 1948. The grants were continued until the late sixties and were a

5 $1,500 for each chronic and convalescent bed.

major factor in making it possible to introduce the hospital insurance and later medical insurance programs across Canada.

Although shortages of beds and personnel were gradually alleviated during the 1950s and Blue Cross, Saskatchewan, British Columbia, Newfoundland and commercial insurance companies all operated efficient hospital insurance plans covering millions of Canadians, there was still room for improvement. In many provinces only a minority of those eligible were insured and the financial problems of hospitals continued.

For these reasons the federal and provincial governments were determined to work out a program of universal hospital insurance. At the 1955 federal-provincial conference and at succeeding meetings the details of what became the Hospital Insurance and Diagnostic Services Act were developed.

The act required that every province wishing federal assistance have legislation providing for the licensure, inspection and supervision of hospitals. Once a province entered the program (supposedly voluntarily, but what provincial government could afford not to enter?) the federal government agreed to pay approximately fifty percent of authorized charges. These included all in-patient, standard, ward costs in active-treatment and convalescent care hospitals as well as hospitals (not nursing homes) for the chronically ill. Tuberculosis and mental institutions were exluded on the grounds that the provinces were already heavily subsidizing these hospitals and a greater priority was put on providing new services rather than rearranging financing of existing ones.

The administration of each plan was left up to each province and the following pattern has emerged. Five provinces (Manitoba, Ontario, Nova Scotia, Alberta, Prince Edward Island) have established a semi-independent commission to administer the insurance plan and in some cases to administer the provincial hospital act. In the other provinces the responsibilities for hospital insurance have been incorporated into the departments of health. In most cases the director of the plan has the status of a deputy minister and whether a 'semi-independent' commission is in effect or not, lines of responsibility go directly to the health minister.

As for benefits provided under the plans, every province, of course, covers all approved and available standard-ward care. Extensive out-patient care has gradually become insured. In Ontario organized home care and nursing-home service (effective 1972) are also provided under the plan. Most provinces provide full out-of-province benefits within Canada or outside North American and lesser coverage for services provided in the United States.

Most provinces have a three-month waiting period before coverage becomes effective as a protective measure. Three provinces – Saskatchewan, Alberta and British Columbia – have deterrent charges of approximately $1 to $2.50 per day for standard-ward care.

All provinces and the Yukon and Northwest Territories finance the insurance plan, at least in part, from general tax revenues. Ontario and Manitoba charge a premium tax and Saskatchewan a hospitalization tax. Coverage is automatic or compulsory in all parts of the country. In provinces with premiums or authorized charges special provision for indigents and welfare recipients has been made.

Since 1959 most provinces had provided a budget-review system whereby each hospital must submit the year's minutely detailed budget well in advance for scrutiny and approval by provincial authorities. If the hospitals could prove the need for the funds then the government provided them. However, by the late sixties it had become clear that despite proven need, some governments simply could not afford to allow hospital costs to climb at such a rapid pace. These provinces then imposed across-the-board maximum rates of expenditure increases.

Concommitant with this new control mechanism, and in some cases partially because of it, there has been a less detailed scrutiny and approval of budget proposals of each hospital so long as the increases fall within provincial guidelines. This type of 'global budgeting' has permitted much greater flexibility for the hospital – a commendable development. The plan also permits more efficient utilization of manpower in the government hospital insurance department.

The government makes payments toward the approved budget of each hospital in regular instalments usually once or twice a month. If there are unforeseen fluctuations in occupancy costs, or other factors that require additional funds, adjustments can occasionally be made in the payments at the time or at year's end when audited financial statements have been prepared.

Some hospitals are allowed to keep part of the differential charges paid for semi-private and private room care. The federal government deducts 50 percent of the differential charges through its share of the insurance costs. In Ontario, Nova Scotia, Newfoundland and Saskatchewan, hospitals can use the entire remainder as surplus revenue. Only in Prince Edward Island and Alberta are differential charges completely deducted from budgeted costs.

All provinces have taken a more active part in capital financing since the introduction of the national health grants in 1948. As construction costs rose dramatically during the 1950s and 1960s the federal grant became increasingly less significant as a portion of the total cost. In the mid-1960s, when the grants were phased out, the federal government was paying only a small part of construction costs in most instances. Only New Brunswick pays 100 percent of hospital construction and renovation costs. Several provinces pay approximately two-thirds of capital costs. In some provinces municipal governments are expected to contribute. Grants vary according to the type of hospital, the highest sums being allocated to teaching and research hospitals. In recent years, even though a government may give full approval to a proposed hospital construction program, the time lag between approval and the actual provision of funds has become increasingly prolonged. New facilities are becoming prohibitively expensive and this factor may dictate a lowered utilization of hospital in-patient facilities.

Over the years many individuals have worked effectively to provide effecient and comprehensive insurance plans. One is reminded of the fine tribute written by Malcolm Taylor:

The most important contribution of all was made by knowledgeable and trained men and women, who were either Blue Cross administrators or hospital leaders. They had helped to mold the plans, fought for comprehensive 'service' benefits and argued for higher premiums to support higher standards and meet increasing costs. In short they were men who had fought for the non-profit, voluntary, humanitarian ideals of the Blue Cross movement. There was unquestionable reluctance on their part to see their projects 'taken over' by the government, but discussions with these leaders suggest that any unhappiness was heavily counterweighed by the knowledge that government action was merely extending to all what they had struggled to bring to many. It was, at once, a tribute to their ideals and an extension of their goals.[6]

RECENT DEVELOPMENTS

Of late the federal and most of the provincial governments have indicated a desire to terminate most of the cost-sharing health grant programs. The federal government would still contribute but on the basis of a per-capita grant with no strings attached. Various authorities, including the personnel of the task forces on the costs of health services, have been concerned for a long time about the lack of flexibility in the insurance grants which prevented provinces from attempting innovations not covered under the Hospital Insurance and Diagnostic Services Act and the Medical Care Act.

6 Malcolm Taylor, 'The Historical Stream,' *Hospitals*, September 16, 1961, p. 122

One of the obvious implications of the new arrangement is that hospitals and various health services will have to compete with other provincial programs for funds from general revenues. No longer will the health field have the benefits of the cost-sharing safeguards ensuring proportionate provincial spending. As a result apprehensions have arisen concerning the intentions of the provinces and about the future of the federal Department of Health. At the end of 1970, federal-provincial discussions were being conducted but no legislative steps had been taken.

Rising costs
Inescapably linked to the problems of hospital financing has been the spectre of rising costs. So serious has this problem become in recent years that the hospital system as we have known it is severely threatened.

Data are not universally available nor reliable before 1930, but the Dominion Bureau of Statistics has estimated that the average rate for public wards was approximately $1.50 per patient per day in 1920. In 1926 it had risen to $1.83 and soared to $1.96 in 1928. My recollection of the twenties in Toronto is that the public-ward rate was $1.50 and then rose to $1.75. The average per diem rate for all patients in active treatment hospitals in 1930, as obtained from the Dominion Bureau of Statistics, was $3.63. Subsequent per diem rates for all patients in such hospitals were $4.74 in 1945, $8.21 in 1950, $21.32 in 1960 and $50.69 in 1970.

In addition to rising rates, patient days have experienced an equally remarkable increase and the total annual cost of providing hospital services has risen from approximately $47 million in the mid-1920s to almost $3 billion in 1970.

Per diem rates have risen for a variety of reasons. A major factor has been the increased complexity and extent of diagnostic and therapeutic services. Hospitals are more comfortable and have many more patient and staff safeguards, all of which add to the cost. But the major cause is the ever increasing payroll, which now makes up from 65 to 75 percent of the annual outlay. For some years many hospitals employed partially recovered patients; sympathetic Sisters in particular often tried to rehabilitate extended-care patients who would never get employment otherwise. Professional personnel, as outlined in the previous chapter, have become more numerous, specialized and highly trained: not only are there more people on the payroll but higher salaries must be paid in accordance with qualifications. Equipment has also increased in cost, and a major portion of this has been due to labour costs.

Other factors relate to hospital management. In the past hospitals have been accused of not always operating in a businesslike manner. To a degree this charge has been true. Many administrators and a proportion of board members have not been experienced businessmen. However, those hospital trustees with corporate experience have found that many features of operating a business cannot be applied to hospitals. If a line of shoes did not prove profitable it was easy to discontinue making or stocking them; a hospital, however, could not discontinue its public wards or its outpatient department because they operated at a loss.

Personnel problems differed too. Layoffs have been almost unknown as hospitals have had to maintain a 'readiness to serve.' On the other hand, hospitals of the past exhibited a cavalier disregard of overtime which makes management today somewhat nostalgic. And, while petty pilfering has existed as in comparable fields of employment, there has been a remarkable degree of honesty at the administrative level in hospitals. In all the years the writer has worked in – and in association with – hospitals, he can number on the fingers of one hand the instances of embezzlement or serious theft. Only one of these cases resulted in a prison sentence. What other field as extensive as hospital administration can boast such a record?

In the past twenty years standardized business methods in hospitals have become widespread. Conventions and the excellent hospital literature have spread the adoption of recognized and efficient procedure. Government regulations and supervision and the use of CHAM, the standard hospital accounting manual, have helped to improve accounting and statistical analysis. In recent years the Dominion Bureau of Statistics (Statistics Canada)-Canadian Hospital Association hospital information system has published, on a quarterly basis, key indices of hospital performance which facilitate comparative analyses. A hospital should be aware of how it deviates from service and costs norms and be able to justify it in the mind of its board. Administrators and their assistants are more thoroughly trained, as are government employees who analyze and approve hospital expenditures. Management and hospital consultants are extensively employed to devise efficient administrative programs for hospitals. Regional planning and centralized services are slowly becoming more extensive.

A further factor accounting for the rise in prices has, of course, been the general rise in the cost of living. Comparisons between the buying power of the 1920 and 1970 dollars are, at best, approximate. Suffice it to say that inflation at an average annual rate of 2 to 3 percent has greatly deflated the value of the currency over these fifty years.

As for the increased numbers of patient days, the influences at work have been fairly clearcut. In 1920, the public attitude toward hospitals as a desirable haven for treatment and cure, rather than the traditional antechamber to the tomb, was just becoming entrenched. Higher standards were being introduced and people were, for the first time, convinced of the advantages of modern medicine as practised in hospitals.

Furthermore, income was rising and many families were able to afford needed hospitalization. Government assistance programs augmenting personal income (as well as those sponsoring hospitalization for indigents) helped to some extent.

The removal of economic barriers through hospital and medical insurance programs has been an important, but not crucial, factor. Critics have claimed for a long time that one of the undesirable side effects of health insurance is that it ensures that utilization of health resources will exceed the real need. To some extent this has proven true; with this fact in mind, those sponsoring insurance plans have demanded controls to make certain that patients claiming coverage have received or are receiving required treatment only. Admission sheets and long-stay forms for each patient certifying that the type of hospital care being given is medically necessary are now required by every provincial hospital insurance plan. Admission for diagnostic reasons have been restricted if the diagnoses can adequately be performed elsewhere.

The population of Canada has more than doubled from 1920 to 1970 and the supply of hospital beds has increased even more – from 77,000 in 1929 to 212,000 in 1970. Although it would be ridiculous to claim that the supply of beds creates the need for them, it does seem to encourage demand. No matter how many beds become available in most communities, the demand for them (as opposed to need) seems to be insatiable. The attitude of the public which has come to expect top quality health care as its right has contributed to this demand. The most important factors, however, are the attitudes and patterns of practice of physicians. It is, after all, the doctor who decides to treat a patient in the hospital rather than at home or in the office – a decision which may involve non-medical as well as strictly medical considerations.

A factor which has tended to reduce the number of patient days in hospitals has been the declining average length of stay in hospital for many diseases due to improved treatment procedures. Also, better ambulatory and home-care services have permitted earlier discharge in many instances. Of course there are some conditions such as various forms of cancer, cystic fibrosis, multiple sclerosis and others, which require more days of care per patient because life expectancy has been prolonged considerably. Improved facilities for the convalescent and chronically ill has enabled physicians to refer more patients to these less expensive hospitals.

Similarly, universal comprehensive medical insurance should lessen the demand for non-surgical beds in active treatment hospitals. Medicare also removes the financial barrier of low-income persons to obtain early medical attention, thereby reducing the need for hospitalization in some cases.

One of the major weaknesses of the existing plans is the lack of incentive for doctors and other health workers not to over-utilize expensive hospital resources. In a few provinces hospitals are allowed to keep some or all of surplus revenues if they are able to operate under budget. However, doctors are the prime determiners of hospital utilization and unless this incentive can be passed onto them its effect will be negligible. It is interesting to note that in some health insurance plans in the United States, notably those of Kaiser-Permanente in California and Health Insurance Plan in New York, the number of patient days in hospital per thousand of insured population is less than half that of most of the Canadian provinces. In these United States plans the doctors work on a contract basis and can retain their pro-rated savings in the overall budget. As far as is discernible the increased use of out-patient facilities, home-care services, group practice clinics and other non-hospital usages, subsequently minimizing the need for in-patient care, has not adversely affected the health of the people.

For many years hospitals were built for $5,000 per bed and less. Today costs have soared to more than $50,000 per bed. This exorbitant figure is prohibitive to all but the most wealthy and desperate. For the most part these prices are beyond the control of the hospital experts but nevertheless they present a real threat to the continued existence of the active treatment hospital as we know it.

For most of the period since 1920 concerned persons have been preoccupied with using the principles of insurance to spread the costs of hospital care from the individual to society as a whole. Today society, reeling under increased taxation in every area of life, is beginning to question whether we can afford our present health delivery system. The federal task forces as well as the provincial governments have shown more than casual interest in the problem.

The stop-gap, arbitrary ceilings on hospital budget increases or moratoriums on construction ordered by the provincial authorities are unsatisfactory for a variety of reasons, the most important of which is that hospitals may have to sacrifice some programs or services. In fact, the greatest danger facing the health field in Canada is that standards of care will be sacrificed in the search for efficiencies. It is crucial to remember that while a nation's wealth is a prime determinant of the state of its health, the converse relationship is also generally true. From a purely economic viewpoint (not to mention the humanitarian and social benefits involved) good health is a bargain at almost any price.

The effect of increased government participation
Since the second world war hospitals have moved on from the time-honoured stance of rugged individualism with only an 'assist' now and then from the government into a new relationship – a partnership – which has had a more fundamental effect on hospitals and their operation than may be recognized easily.

The partnership was inevitable. For many decades we have been moving inexorably towards more state participation in so many of our essential services. We have seen this steadily increasing assumption of government control in the railways, in wire and wireless communication, in power production and in other systems and services. A large number of other businesses and business systems have not been taken over but have been heavily subsidized. We see industries and groups paid to produce – or paid *not* to. It seems, too, that most other endeavours are surrounded by a forest of restrictions, most of which we have clamored for ('There ought to be a law against ... !') and then criticize when a slow-moving state puts them in force. Leaders in democracies are sensitive to the ballot and are inclined to be more swayed by pressure groups than by the unorganized majority. The whole trend is towards more state participation – 'creeping socialism' or 'galloping socialism' depending upon your political viewpoint.

The partnership with hospitals was inevitable from a financial viewpoint also. Philanthropy has taken a beating with soaring corporation and personal taxes. With the growth of welfare provisions, supported or heavily subsidized by municipal and government taxation and succession duties, hospital boards have found it exceedingly difficult to raise the necessary funds for hospital expansion or to meet operating deficits. (One wonders what would have happened to our hospital system if substantial government construction grants had not been set up and if hospital insurance had not been developed to take the financial sting out of hospitalization. With costs escalating to astronomical heights our hospitals would have become woefully inadequate and obsolete.)

One cannot but ponder the future course of this partnership. It is not static, bound by legal contract and incorporation papers with a stated division of voting power. This is a flexible, ill-defined relationship, changing all the time and with the state controlling new capital and generally writing the regulations. Definitely it has greatly improved the facilities, plant and staff for serving the patient. Hospital leaders realize that they must have more financial assistance and have repeatedly urged more government support of their programs. But they are concerned that these developments are undermining the concept of voluntary support and service. Not only has voluntary assistance been the backbone of hospital provision for centuries but it has also created an atmosphere of dedication and service which has been of inestimable value to the sick and suffering. Although some parts of Canada, notably the Prairie provinces, are served largely by municipal hospitals, they also have been aided by voluntary groups who have contributed extensively to the welfare and comfort of the patients.

Industry and commerce generally seems to be affected by a blight which has dissipated the employee's interest in his work, reduced his concern for his product, weakened discipline and turned us into a nation of clockwatchers. Anyone who professes or displays a dedication to his work is written off as a 'square.' A few years ago an American psychologist addressed a meeting at the university where I was teaching. His subject was a two-year research program he had completed on the attitudes of employees in a large Chicago hospital. What I remember in particular was the amusement and incredulity he displayed in telling of one employee who had no family connections and therefore volunteered to work on Christmas so that someone else could be off with his family. How foolish can one be? Nor could the psychologist appreciate the motivation of an employee who came back voluntarily on a long holiday weekend to work in the laundry because he knew the nursery would likely be running short of diapers. Apparently concern for others is becoming an evidence of mental aberration.

It is hoped that the hospital will continue to be a centre, even if only an oasis, where voluntary effort will flourish, where the needs of suffering humanity will come first, and where restricted hours of work and detailed limitations of duties will not prove more important than saving the life of a patient.

6

Changes in hospital construction

Another major contribution to improved standards of care and efficiency has been the evolution between 1920 and 1970 of hospital design and construction. Hospital design underwent a number of changes during the 1920s and 1930s but surprisingly few as compared to the alterations since the second world war.

THE PUBLIC WARDS

During the twenties the long corridor-type public wards of twenty or thirty beds common to the larger city hospitals were under attack as unsuitable for optimum patient care. New hospitals built after this time did not include wards larger than six or eight beds. In some older hospitals large wards were broken up into cubicles of four to eight beds.

By today's standards even some of these improvements seem primitive. But it is well to remember that our viewpoint is modified by our position in time. A generation before, a member of my family who was a nurse in the old Toronto General Hospital (when it was located on Gerrard Street East – that is, prior to 1912) used to tell of conditions in the large wards of her time. She told how the nurses would spread sheets of 'tanglefoot' on the patients' beds to catch flies. Window screens were a rarity. She recalled the day when the ward mouser, a long-time unregistered but popular inhabitant of the wing, forgot about the fly-catching ritual and jumped on the bed of one of her favourite patients. By the time the cat finally rolled from the bed she was effectively encased in all four large sheets of flypaper: one baleful eye and the odd paw were the only evidence that the moving apparition was propelled by a cat.

Those days – thank goodness – were long gone before the twenties and the thirties.

The reduction in ward size was not made without some misgivings. The advantages of smaller units were obvious – more privacy, less disturbance at night, better opportunity to minister to the seriously ill, more ease in teaching medical students and an atmosphere more conducive to a higher average occupancy. Despite the advantages it was agreed, however, that the large open wards permitted better supervision, particularly at night when the nursing staff was at a minimum. A common practice was to bring the seriously ill or post-anaesthetic patients close to the nurses' desk in the centre of the large wards where they could be under the nurses' almost constant eye. Other patients would raise the alarm if someone was choking or had fallen out of bed. Up-patients helped the bedridden, saving footsteps for the nurses.

Administrators, concerned with perennial deficits, believed that smaller rooms would add to the cost of running the hospital. Many of the patients themselves *liked* the big wards; there was more sociability and more action all day long. There were other psychological advantages; any patient feeling sorry for himself had only to raise his eyes and see someone else much less fortunate.

However, the trend favored smaller room units and for many years now practically no construction in general hospitals has contained any adult patients' rooms with more than four beds. Convalescent and extended-care institutions have taken longer to give up six- or eight-bed rooms, partly because of the patients' desire for company, but also because of the cost of operation.

Today, more and more emphasis is placed on privacy. This is probably due to several factors: more widespread affluence, the popularity of semi-private Blue Cross coverage and the workmen's compensation provision of semi-private care in most provinces. New construction usually provides for a preponderance of single and two-bed wards with none having more than four beds.

Many planners and architects have prophesied that the hospital of the future will contain single rooms only. I am not so sure but I *can* see it as a possibility *if* general hospital admissions are limited to acutely ill patients only, if practically all diagnostic cases are treated on an ambulatory basis or housed in hostels, and if less acutely ill patients are largely treated under home-care conditions or in less highly equipped institutions.

We are more likely to see the disappearance of the two-bed semi-private room, created to provide 'private' status to the individual of limited means and given a continuing lease on life by Blue Cross, workmen's compensation and various sickness insurance programs. There is little more upsetting to a patient of taste than to be trapped in a hospital room with the second bed occupied by an obnoxious person who smokes incessantly, uses foul language, has endless visitors who sit on one's bed without asking permission, keeps the radio or TV on full blast and snores in three octaves. Studies have shown that the noise and disturbance level is lower in a four-bed room than it is in a two-bed room, possibly because of the larger size and the helpful distraction of other sounds and activities.

My own prediction is that we are likely to find hospitals evolving towards single and four-bed rooms only.

CONSOLIDATION OF BUILDINGS

The most noticeable change in the thirties and forties was a tendency to consolidate the various hospital buildings. The 'pavilion' style of construction had been popular in Europe for many years and the concept had been accepted here by many of our larger hospitals. When studying at the Allgemeine Krankenhaus in Vienna in 1926, I was intrigued to note the miniature railway which ran from building to building transporting supplies and bulk containers of cooked food. These containers and articles were lifted by hand out of the little open rail cars and carried up the steps into the buildings. All of this took time but help was cheap and it was undoubtedly an effective means of transport between the various buildings of a spread-out institution. In Canada, a separate building was sometimes erected to house a specialized service, such as the Montreal Neurological Institute at the Royal Victoria Hospital in Montreal. Frequently the obstetrical unit – as the Ross Pavilion in the same hospital, or the Burnside Pavilion at the Toronto General Hospital – was housed in a separate building.

There was a good reason for this pavilion-style of construction, for the sulfa drugs and the antibiotics had not been developed and puerperal sepsis was a tragic sword of Damocles hanging over every young mother. Dr Roger de Lee of Chicago, a leading obstetrician of the first world war period and author of the text book which was our bible in midwifery, thundered on every possible occasion that obstetrical patients always should be housed in a separate building.

Changing procedures in hospitals created new problems. Patients became more mobile and went to treatment rather than having treatment coming to them. They went to X-ray, to the laboratories, to isolation, to certain equipment located in the out-patient department, to intensive care, to the operating rooms, or to physical therapy. Centralized food service meant trundling heavy food trucks from the kitchen to the patient floors; central sterilizing, mobile laundry shelf-trucks, and oxygen tents from the inhalation therapy department meant more trucking. Patients found themselves visited by seemingly endless successions of laboratory technicians, assistant dietitians, office personnel, heating adjusters, electronics repair men, research fellows, research statisticians and countless more. All of this increased activity called for shorter lines of communication; time spent in walking or pushing equipment along corridors meant more and more dollars as labour costs rose, dollars spent only peripherally in health care.

The result was the widespread adoption of the 'monolithic' hospital as contrasted to the 'pavilion' type. Typical examples were the Montreal General Hospital, the Victoria General in Halifax, the Saint John General Hospital, the Calgary General, Ste Sacrement and the Jeffrey Hale's Hospital in Quebec City and the University Hospital in Saskatoon. Some hospitals were too big to begin with to make the transition in one step; examples would be the two largest – the Vancouver General Hospital and the Toronto General Hospital. Others have added large units but have not been able, for good financial reasons, to abandon serviceable pavilion-units immediately. Examples would be the Kingston General Hospital, the University Hospital in Edmonton, the Hamilton General Hospital, the Winnipeg General Hospital and the Victoria Hospital in London. Some still preferred to keep obstetrics separate, such as the Royal Jubilee in Victoria and the Winnipeg General.

The transition to the monolithic hospital, when a new structure was added to the old, created a problem. The buildings dating back to the early years usually had ceilings as high as fourteen or sixteen feet. This height was necessary for ventilation before artificially induced air movement was developed. Now a nine- or ten-foot ceiling is considered adequate, with a lower ceiling in corridors to accommodate major pipes. This disparity between the old and new ceiling heights has required ramps to connect adjacent floor levels, and sometimes has resulted in no through connection on an upper floor. Ramps are always a problem where there is movement of patients or corridor-borne supplies. The only practical solution has been to accept ramps as a necessary but temporary evil until the existing older buildings can be replaced with modern ones. The situation has not been helped by a common earlier idea that the main entrance should only be reached by a formidable flight of outdoor steps. Now the main floor is usually only one to four feet above ground level, depending upon the terrain, and usually with all but one step inside the building protected from the weather.

Within another decade or two I expect practically all of these ramps and high staircases will disappear as new buildings replace the old. If government assistance for replacement of obsolete buildings is again intensified, their disappearance would be materially hastened.

It should be noted that Europe and Great Britain have also moved in this direction. At the 1937 meeting of the (then) International Hospital Association in Paris, Hjalmar Cedarstrom, the eminent Swedish hospital architect, created much interest with his plans for the Soder Hospital near Stockholm, a long spine with numerous cross wings for patients, planned on the principle of a wire tie-holder. The Birmingham Hospital, built in Captain J.E. Stone's time, was another example of this consolidated planning.[1] Now nearly all of the new construction in Britain and Europe follows this general pattern.

REARRANGEMENT OF SERVICES

In the early decades of the fifty-year period we are examining hospitals were laid out much differently from today.

In the twenties and thirties almost all hospitals had the operating suite on the top floor, with the operating rooms themselves placed to take advantage of the north light. The top floor was selected for the operating suite partly to gain the advantage of skylight and vertical windows, but also to achieve the greatest distance from street dust. Obstetrics was usually on the floor below the operating rooms and often with a nearly identical floor plan.

The emergency department and out-patient department were usually located in the basement. In the basement, too, were radiology and pathology. These latter two departments were relative newcomers to the hospital and were shoved in wherever space could be found.

The laundry was usually located atop the boiler house which was often some distance from the hospital proper. This placement created the usual problem of getting clean laundry across the intervening space in rainy weather, or through a dark, hot, low-ceilinged pipe tunnel.

The isolation ward was usually far down a basement corridor, alarm-

---

1 In Britain in the thirteenth century St. Tomas', one of the royal hospitals, was built as a series of enclosed courts, all connected into one elongated building.

ingly free of any personnel through the long night. If the number of patients or the severity of their illness did not warrant the posting of a nurse, one could be summoned – it was hoped – by the ringing of a bell or by telephone.

Today the arrangement is quite different. For years surgeons have preferred to operate by artificial light at all times. Operating room windows – if there are any – are never opened so street dust is no problem. The operating suite can be, and is, located anywhere within the hospital. And so with the delivery suite.

The trend has been to have the clinical-service units clustered in one area to facilitate the movement of personnel and equipment. This developed slowly. A common arrangement about the time of the second world war and for some years later was to develop a service building central to the patient wings. In simplified form the service building would be the stem of a 'T' with the patients in the crossbar. A typical vertical arrangement was a combination of clinical and domestic services:

Top floor	Operative suite (still unchanged)
Third floor	Delivery suite
Second floor	Laboratory and X-ray
Main floor	Administrative, business and nursing offices (possibly chapel), doctors' facilities and medical records
Basement or ground	Emergency, outpatient, kitchen, dining, stores

This arrangement simplified the architectural planning for it took the atypical floors out of the patients' wings and permitted more specialized structural and service features. It did not, however, solve the problem of obtaining a more efficient functional arrangement.

In the late fifties and early sixties it became apparent that the various clinical services should be grouped even more closely together. Moreover the service wing idea was proving inadequate because some services (like pathology and radiology) were rapidly outgrowing others, making floor assignments unrealistic. Nor was it practical, with increasing out-patient treatment, to have radiology and pathology located on an upper floor as was often the case.

Out of this situation came the 'pad-and-towers' concept. A base, frequently containing a basement and main floor, but sometimes more storeys, and criss-crossed with corridors, covered a large area; above this base or pad rose one or more towers of patients' floors.

The base contained all of the clinical services which logic demands should be together – emergency department, out-patient clinics, radiology, pathology, operative suite, pharmacy, physical medicine, special investigative laboratories and, sometimes, the cancer unit. These services were grouped together on one or two floors. Elsewhere in the pad were located the dietary department, stores and the receiving entrance. Administration offices, business offices, medical records, doctors' facilities, housekeeping, laundry and employees' facilities were also located in the base. These facilities were grouped and related to each other on a functional basis and also to the various entrances.

The arrangement has proven very satisfactory. With the increasing amount of emergency work it is advantageous to have available immediately not only the X-ray and the laboratory but also the facilities of the main operative suite. With modern lighting and ventilation, it is possible to use inside space for a wide variety of functions. Actually this pad-and-towers concept has been used by large hotels for many years with full street frontage of the hotel used for stores and restaurants; above these service outlets extend the wings of guests' rooms.

The pad-and-tower concept has one design drawback, however. If the patient towers were high-rise, the required supporting columns severely restricted the use of the space in the base beneath. It was impossible, for instance, to include an auditorium or large lecture theatre. During the sixties even this problem was solved – where the site was sufficiently large, the architects began to shift the patient towers to one side of the service base. Thus, no ponderous supporting columns obstructed the open space of the pad. Service functions and even auditoriums could be freely placed in the base pad and later renovations were more easily made.

(In somewhat analogous fashion, many post-second world war churches moved the traditional steeple from atop the church building to its side, retaining the symbolic function but removing the structural support from within the building.)

In a sense, this new design concept was a return to the old idea of keeping the service wing separate from the patient wings. In this instance, though, the services are arranged horizontally rather than vertically as before.

THE DOUBLE CORRIDOR

An innovation of the second world war period that seems to have become a permanent feature of planning is the double corridor. This idea was developed by the late Charles F. Neergaard of New York City, a hospital consultant who made many contributions to the functional planning of hospitals.[2]

The double corridor consisted of two corridors (rather than one) running the length of the wing. Patient rooms are located on the outside of each corridor and the various service facilities such as nurses' station, utilities, diet kitchen, stairway, and so forth occupied the space between the halls. Advantages to this plan, as compared to the conventional single corridor plan included:

1
A 30 percent saving in length of each patient wing over the single-corridor plan still accommodating the same number of patients.
2
With shorter wing lengths, there is less perimeter devoted to any given number of patients, hence less heat loss during winter, and less strain on air conditioning in summer.
3
The building would be eighty-five or more feet wide; the single-corridor building is usually fifty or fifty-two feet wide and much less in older buildings. The extra width permits infinitely better layouts for operative suites, delivery suites, radiology, the laboratories, emergency, dietary, physical therapy and other departments.
4
All of the outside walls can be devoted to patient space. In single-corridor design much valuable outside wall space is given over to service rooms.
5
Every patient, including the most remote, is much closer to the nurses' station.
6
With two corridors, patients requiring two kinds of treatment can be housed on the same floor. Thus, children and adults can be cared for on the same floor as can obstetric and surgical patients.

The double corridor is now used across Canada and around the world. With the development of the pad-and-tower concept, multiple-corridor plans were evolved, five or six in parallel. The square plan, of practical use

2 It was my privilege to have been a partner of Neergaard in the (then) hospital consulting firm of Neergaard, Agnew and Craig from 1950 until Mr Neergaard's retirement a few years before his death in 1961. It was a delightful experience to work with this capable, forceful, big-hearted but irascible redheaded dynamo to whom the best solution was never good enough.

for office units and certain clinics, is really just a shortened double corridor.

The double corridor was not accepted overnight. Many architects opposed it. They objected: 'It is wide and looks dumpy compared to the long, narrow single corridor.' 'It requires 15 percent more corridor space.' (This 'criticism' was quite true, but corridor space is comparatively inexpensive and the cost is more than balanced by not having to heat the core rooms as would be the case if they were on an outside wall.) 'The core rooms must have artificial ventilation.' (All new construction today utilizes controlled ventilation so this objection has lost its point.) An objection of some hospital designers, that nurses had to go around the core to get supplies or perform tasks, would have been true only through a failure to put enough cross-corridors through the core.

There are still occasions when the single-corridor plan seems to work best, particularly in connecting units. However, the double corridor is one of the major planning advances of the fifty-year period we are studying.

THE ROUND HOSPITAL

A diversion of the fifties and early sixties was the rise and fall of the enthusiasm for the round hospital. This design placed the nurses' station at the centre of a circle and the patients' rooms on the circumference. An early experimental unit of some twelve beds at the Methodist Hospital in Rochester, Minnesota, had some excellent attributes. The nurses in the centre had a direct view of every patient, the distance to any room was minimal and the patients were pleased to be under such close surveillance. Publicity led to widespread interest by architects and numerous hospitals were built, some in large circles containing as many as forty or fifty patients. Others were built with a group of smaller round units connected by corridors or arms. The idea was elaborated for larger circles to include operative suites, emergency departments and other units with odd-shaped rooms and confusing sub-corridors.

The original idea was excellent for an intensive care unit of not more than twelve to fifteen patients where constant oversight is desirable. However, this constant central oversight was frequently disrupted by trips to a connecting arm where equipment was stored. To build a whole hospital of small circular units, difficult to supervise, was not practical. To create larger units raised the difficulty of an enlarged core, for the encircling corridor, naturally, had to keep within a bedroom width of the external wall. This was apparent in the interesting design for a forty-eight bed circle in the Cabrini Hospital in Montreal, where the large internal core contained various rooms for utilities, treatment and laundry, a stairway and two nurses' stations, each to serve half of the patients on the floor. With the ability of the nurses to observe patients directly reduced to a few rooms only, and with most of the patients further than a corridor-width away, the round hospital lost much of its value. Moreover, most of the rooms had waste space in the angles of little practical use despite some ingenious planning.

THE OPERATIVE SUITE

This department has seen remarkable change since the first world war.

Size
In the early years of our fifty-year study period most Canadian hospitals had small operating rooms – small by the standards of today. Many were less than 300 square feet in area and some as small as 275 square feet and less. In some, the scrub-up sinks were located within the operating room, a practice frowned on even then. (It was accepted as necessary in the emergency operating room but discouraged in the main operating suite.) Supplies, sterile and others, were often kept on shelving within the operating room. As new equipment was developed and improved it crowded the small operating rooms even more. As nitrous oxide came into general use as an anaesthetic, the bulky equipment it required had to be provided for. Pedestal lamps, often with a bulky battery in the base, took up more precious floor space. As blood transfusions became common during surgery, the equipment proliferated.

Larger operating rooms were obviously necessary. Rooms of 320 to 340 square feet became common. These larger rooms were considered 'major' operating rooms. Smaller operating rooms were used for the 'minor' surgery required in such techniques as tonsillectomies, cystoscopy and so forth. By the time of the second world war, operating rooms of 340 square feet were common. By the 1950s, a size of 360 square feet was considered optimum and by the sixties most hospital consultants were providing for operating rooms of 400 square feet. As sophisticated equipment increased in availability, the operating room grew to accommodate it.

In the late sixties, with the development of open-heart surgery with its massive assemblage of equipment and supplementary personnel, hospitals specializing in this and cranial surgery found they required operating rooms of 500 to 600 square feet. Except for these 'jumbo' rooms, the trend since the mid-forties has been to make all operating rooms of the same size, 'minor' rooms distinctive only in that they contain less equipment. Sometimes the rooms primarily for endoscopy have been kept to smaller proportions.

Location

As previously mentioned, operating rooms were traditionally placed on the hospital's top floor to take full advantage of the sunless north light combined with an overhead skylight, and to get the maximum distance from street dust, a consideration when operating room windows often had to be kept open (although usually screened). With the development of air-conditioning, artificial light and ventilation, the operative suite was freed from its fixed location and could be placed in a hospital design where it made most sense. As functional relationships came to dominate hospital planning, it finally came to rest near emergency, the laboratories, radiology, and the other clinical services – usually on one of the lower floors.

Ancillary Facilities

The operative suite is several times larger now than at the beginning of this fifty-year period. This results not only from the increased size of the operating rooms themselves, but also from the inclusion of many ancillary areas. These include offices and a workroom for the anaesthetists;[3] supervisors' office; holding space for patients awaiting surgery; a 'quick section' room; teaching space for medical students, student nurses or operating room technicians; doctors' and nurses' changing rooms; a recovery room; a coffee area and special stretcher parking area. With greater width of buildings, corridors can be wider. Most of the better-planned hospitals have a peripheral corridor leading to the operating rooms as well as an internal corridor; thus 'clean' traffic is separated from contaminated traffic and patient traffic from service traffic.

Observation Facilities

From the 1930s to the 1950s a number of hospitals built one- or two-row observation galleries high on a lateral wall. Observation was through glass, frequently aided by 'intercom' equipment. These galleries were a great

3 In Canada, except in very few instances, the anaesthetists are licensed members of the medical profession, in larger centres almost invariably certified as specialists. In the United States a high proportion of the anaesthetics are given by specially trained nurses called 'anesthetists.' The medical specialists in anaesthesiology are known as 'anesthesiologists.'

improvement over the old 'pipes,' a movable two-level stand constructed of piping at the side of the operating room (and from which vantage point we students saw practically nothing of interest except the occasional wink from a masked nurse.) Furthermore, it was much safer for the patient than having a visitor breathing down the neck of the surgeon as he worked.

Even observation galleries are being relegated to the past as more of our teaching (and other large) hospitals install closed-circuit television. This permits the observers, frequently in a room elsewhere in the hospital, to get a view of the operative field as good as that of the surgeons. In the new operating rooms at the Toronto General Hospital, for instance, the observers look down through sloping glass from a circular gallery directly overhead. In case their vision is restricted by a surgeon's head or distance, they can turn to a small television screen beside them for close-up details.

Lighting
Lighting within the operative suite has steadily improved. Some surgeons, it is recalled, were reluctant to give up natural lighting during daylight hours; a simple spotlight was considered by them to be adequate to find a recalcitrant fallopian tube or a shy gallbladder. The French Scialitique overhead light was the most popular type in the 1920s, replacing earlier installations that were frequently single lights with small reflectors mounted on rectangular piping above the table. Other low-heat shadowless models shared the market. The Hallothane light, made up of a large number of ceiling-installed refracting glass squares, focused batteries of lights on the operating area; the angles of the beams of light could be controlled in the larger installations by a panel of switches. Twin clusters of overhead lights on parallel rails were yet to come. The egg-shaped ceiling and walls, dotted with spotlights, were introduced in Europe in such well-known hospitals as St Lô in France and the Western General in Edinburgh, but still have not become popular in America.

By the late forties artificial light had taken over the operating room almost entirely. As we have seen, the grouping of functionally similar services permitted operating rooms to be placed anywhere – even in the interior of a building without an outside wall. By the sixties, most operative suites were without windows except, perhaps, for a high strip window to provide clean-up lighting. Some of us, in our advisory capacity to hospitals, have seen a danger here, especially for the nurses who work long hours in this windowless environment. The cillary muscles of the eye are at rest only when the eye is focused at infinity. In a closed space these muscles are constantly under tension and, if continued for hours, day after day, systemic reaction could occur. In one hospital I know of the operating room windows were replaced by glass bricks – a logical arrangement. Shortly after the substitution a number of the operating room staff began to complain of headaches. The ophthalmologist on the staff quietly arranged for a cluster of glass bricks in each room to be replaced by clear glass, so that the nurses could see the treetops and clouds. Within days the headaches disappeared.

Operating tables and service outlets
The better operating tables, capable of many adjustments, came into more general use in the 1930s. In the thirties, too, we began to see floor outlets for suction, nitrous oxide and oxygen. Most of these installations were mounted on a base about six inches in height. This arrangement had some advantage over the wall outlets then being experimented with, for it did away with the tubes or 'spaghetti' on the floor. There was the disadvantage, however, that the position of the table became fixed, which made it difficult to focus the light for certain operations. Also personnel sometimes tripped over the low base if the table were moved. Some hospitals raised the base to a height or 24 to 30 inches to minimize this possibility.

Later came ceiling outlets over the head of the operating table. These installations became more elaborate as the surgeon wanted a separate suction outlet when compressed air was required to operate bone drills and other equipment. In the fifties it became routine to install two banks of ceiling outlets over diagonally opposite corners of the table, partly to permit re-positioning of the table and partly to provide separate outlets for the surgeon. Problems have arisen when mobile ceiling lights – especially twin lights on rails – have fouled these ceiling outlets. Sometimes there is conflict with down-draft outlets for conditioned ventilation. These usually result from lack of co-ordinated planning and need not occur.

Emergency lighting has always been necessary for, in the earlier decades of electric power usage, cutoffs were frequent and sometimes disastrously lengthy. Winter blizzards played havoc with surgery (and hospital operation *in toto*). As the utility companies provided more adequate and prompt service, the hospitals depended more and more upon electrical power for nearly every activity including general heating. In some cases even the shortest breaks became serious, as, for instance, in an interruption of the 'iron lung' around a polio victim or the halting of an elevator containing a woman in labor.

At first hospitals supplemented the ubiquitous flashlight with wall-mounted battery lights and battery-in-base floor lights in the operating and delivery rooms. Some hospitals installed diesel-fired auxiliary generators to supply emergency power to certain rooms and corridors and one elevator. Emergency generators were not common until the power inadequacies in industrial areas during the second world war led to a general provision of auxiliary power generators. Oddly enough, although many hospitals were thus enabled during power failures to activate one of the elevators, I never found a hospital (on somewhat routine enquiry) which instructed its personnel which elevator to use for obstetrical patients going to the delivery room or for patients returning from surgery. Frequently only the engineer seemed to know which elevator was working.

In more recent years, generators with much greater capacity have been installed, some able almost to duplicate the normal requirements for lighting and power. Where possible hospitals now receive their normal electrical supply from two sources, thus minimizing cutoff from a strictly local cause.

Electro-static hazards
These have been a constant concern to hospitals. Tragic explosions have taken the lives of patients and staff. The situation has been more serious in the central part of Canada with its dry winter weather than on the two coasts where the climate is more moist. We have tried many preventive measures – conductive flooring of many types; conductive casters on operating tables and conductive soles and bootees to ground personnel; Horton inter-couplers to connect equipment; conductive gloves for anaesthesiologists; equipment to raise the humidity in the room to at least 55 RH (rate of humidity), no easy accomplishment in sub-zero prairie weather; the banishment of any electric-motor apparatus in the area; explosion-proof switches; and many other precautions. Despite every effort, explosions still have occurred, although much less frequently. Usually the explosion has been traced to some inadequacy, either in the grounding of a piece of equipment or to some slight oversight on the part of an individual.

In the sixties many operating rooms were designed around the research then taking place in the non-explosive anaesthetics. As we enter the seventies, the confidence in non-explosive anaesthetics seems to have been well founded. But time alone will tell decisively.

While attention here has been focused on preventive measures in the operative suite, comparable problems were being encountered in those emergency departments where general anaesthetics were permitted. In many (usually smaller) hospitals, for instance, it was customary to set fractures under general anaesthetic in the radiological department. The principles of control have been broadly similar and it is hoped that the ultimate solution can be the same – non-explosive anaesthetics.

AIR CLIMATIZATION

I could have used the term 'climate control', or 'environmental control.' ('Air-conditioning' has been so long synonymous with 'air-cooling' that I have avoided the term as ambiguous.) Great change and development have occurred over this half century.

Natural ventilation was the *only* ventilation in the twenties and thirties. All patients' rooms had windows that could be opened and so did the operative and delivery suites until well into the thirties. I have seen, in some hospitals, a sterile sheet laid over the instrument table until the operation would begin. At times a fine cinder dust from the nearby smoke stack was clearly visible. It was probably less a hazard to the patient than the inadequate (if any) mask worn by the surgeon. In hot weather electric fans were placed in the patients' rooms, in offices and elsewhere. In most locations – particularly in radiology and the kitchen – the fans were acceptable, indeed often considered a luxury. But frequently they were used in the operating room and the delivery room, where they created both a bacterial and an electrostatic hazard; in the laboratory, too, they created a potential hazard.

As window air coolers came into general use in the 1940s and early 1950s, many were used in hospital offices, radiology, dining rooms and various other locations. They were used also in operating and delivery rooms to some extent but, by this time, with an increased awareness of their explosion potential if they were less than five feet above the floor. They were not routinely installed in patients' rooms but a number of hospitals had several rooms equipped with window conditioners primarily for the use of obese cardiac patients and others needing this facility. (Perhaps there were not more because most patients did not like the constant noise the early machines generated.)

But what was a luxury in the forties became looked upon as a necessity in the fifties. Air-cooled operating and delivery rooms became a necessity. In the southern and central states completely 'air-conditioned' hospitals (basically air-cooled) became accepted as normal and, by the early 1960s, many new hospitals in the warmer parts of Canada became fully air-cooled too.

For many decades most larger hospitals had systems of air removal by natural or fan-induced currents through outlets on the roof. These systems were usually inadequate, producing far below the necessary rate of room air replacement. Even into the sixties many hospitals still suffered an inadequate supply of replacement air. Some still depend on inlets too close to ground level and some have roof inlets too close to the exhaust outlets.

In the late twenties and early thirties air humidification began to receive more attention. This new concern was due, in part, to a realization that an RH 55 was necessary in the operating room in very cold dry weather to prevent static sparks. Some children's hospitals installed high-humidity rooms to replace the familiar steam kettle to aid patients with respiratory difficulties. In the early thirties it was recognized that nurseries for the newborn, too, should have a higher-than-usual RH.

In the forties attention focused on ways to reduce the bacterial content of the air being channelled to various departments. It began to be realized, too, that the re-circulation of untreated air was not without danger. The re-circulation of air, planned originally to economize by reducing the loss of heat, resulted in an amazingly rapid spread of bacteria throughout the hospital. Experimental testing with readily recognized but harmless strains of bacteria proved the point beyond any doubt.

Out of all this developed a number of systems of ventilation, directing currents by slight degrees of positive or negative pressure so as to ensure the right type of air for operating or delivery rooms, or for special rooms for burn cases with large areas of vulnerable skin surface. The air is washed and sterilized by various means, humidified in varying degrees for different areas and heated or cooled as required. Each improvement has required other changes. Windows are permanently closed, sometimes a psychologically difficult condition for older patients to accept. In addition to their value in fire control, the closed stairwells, elevator shafts, and frequent in-corridor doors required by law also serve to keep the air-pressure controls and planned airflows in proper balance.

BUILDING CODES

The diversity of building codes was a real problem for hospital planners through the early part of this half-century; indeed, it remains a very real problem today. Provincial requirements vary widely in depth of detail and local requirements vary from no control at all to a degree of conservatism which practically rules out some promising new building materials and economic methods of construction.

In 1938 Major-General A.G.L. McNaughton, president of the National

Research Council, announced that the council, in collaboration with the dominion fire commission and the dominion housing administration, was undertaking the preparation of a model building code for Canada with the intent of bringing some order into the existing unsatisfactory situation. The Canadian Hospital Council was asked to name representatives to the NRC advisory committee and Rev Father Verreault, then president, appointed James Govan of Govan, Ferguson and Lindsay, one of Canada's leading firms of hospital architects, A.J. Swanson, chairman of the CHC committee on construction, and myself as hospital planning representatives.

I have already spoken of Arthur Swanson. 'Jimmy' Govan was a short, slight Scotsman, bursting with energy and sprouting ideas in an endless supply. During the twenties and thirties, he and his associates planned more hospitals in Canada than any other architectural firm. He was particularly innovative in such areas as heat insulation and fire control.

The research council's committee made a great deal of progress and eventually produced a suggested national building code that including zoning requirements, classification of occupancies, wood construction, wind and snow loads, fire protection, live and dead loads, excavations, foundations and sanitation requirements.

RADIO INTERFERENCE

Technical progress is seldom achieved without some repercussions. We have always been appreciative of the continuing improvement of safety in air travel. Improved air-safety measures have been costly to hospitals near airports, however.

I shall use the Royal Alexandra Hospital in Edmonton to illustrate my point. For years planes landed and took off from this airport just beyond the hospital. (I am speaking of the old hospital across the road from the new complex.) A Trans-Canada Airlines (Air Canada) pilot once told me that he and other pilots would 'draw a bead' on one of the red warning lights that marked the hospital roof and try to come as close as they could to the light without hitting it. In doing so they were in perfect alignment with the runway. What it did to the nerves of personnel and patients just a few feet beneath that roof would be another story.

In a later day, with more sophisticated radio control of air traffic, the occasional interference by hospital emanations became a serious matter to pilots and ground control. In 1938 the Department of Transport began to warn hospitals that their electric equipment – particularly electrotherapy and some radiological installations – was seriously interfering with air-traffic control. The department delayed action as long as possible but continued complaints from many parts of Canada eventually necessitated action.

For some months radiation-free equipment had been available so that the enforced regulation, when it came in 1942, was neither unexpected nor too costly to implement.

FUTURE PLANNING

Hospital planning of the future must provide more flexibility. The obvious goal should be a comparatively permanent outer shell and an interior structure that can be altered extensively – and as often as necessary – at a minimum cost in a minimum of time. The modern, rigidly framed, fire-resistant structure should be usable for at least seventy-five years – maybe more. Many of today's hospitals are now functionally obsolete in twenty-five to thirty years, yet continue in use at an escalating operational cost because of the expense of razing and replacing.

Some efforts have been made to meet this need of flexibility. Plumbing has been concentrated, where possible, on the corridor side of rooms. In laboratories and offices, removable side walls have been used; these are usually of metal and do permit more flexibility but also permit more sound transmission than tile or stud-and-plaster walls. In recent years extensive stretches of open space are achieved by special engineering and these spaces can be partitioned with light, non-weight-bearing walls that are easily and simply shifted about. (One example of such planning is the McMaster University Medical School in Hamilton, Ontario.)

Two other building trends which have radically altered some aspects of the construction industry have had little impact on hospitals as yet: I refer to the use of prefabricated building parts and the use of standardized plans.

The use of prefabricated building parts, constructed in some central location and assembled on the site, has been amply proven as a means of holding the line on ever-climbing building costs. (Perhaps the most dramatic use of prefabricated materials – though *not* of its low cost – was at 'Habitat' at Expo '67 in Montreal.) For some reason, the use of prefabricated building parts has never become widespread in the building of Canadian hospitals.

In England, though, the Oxford Regional Hospital Board, working closely with the architects, engineers and fabricators, has developed an 'Oxford Method' of construction based upon a four-inch module and a two-foot planning grid; prefabrication of lightweight materials and rapid assembly are part of the concept.[4] Various modules varying up to twenty-four or thirty-six inches have been proposed from time to time but adoption has been slow.

This approach to overcoming the steadily rising cost of construction has been paralleled over the years by the concept of standard plans for hospitals of various sizes and types. As long as the writer can remember, this proposal has popped up periodically. There has been much to commend it, too, for it is exceedingly slow to work out all of the innumerable details for every hospital construction job, making every one custom built. Yet the more one becomes familiar with the physical requirements of hospitals the more obvious it becomes that practically every hospital must provide features unique to its own needs, or, more specifically, to the needs of its key medical staff members who determine what type of work and what procedures must be provided for. Standard plans have worked fairly well in the army and the Canadian Red Cross tried them out years ago with some of its outpost hospitals. The concept might be adopted with reasonable success with completely new hospitals but would fail entirely in the case of additions. Our own experience as consultants in more than 700 planning projects indicates how rarely expansion or renovation undertakings are similar – and they far outnumber the total of completely new hospitals. Moreover, using stock plans from a dusty file greatly reduces the amount of innovation and adaptation to new concepts so essential to progress.

What I foresee is a 'middle of the road' development, the utilization of more modular design and prefabrication to combat rising costs, with a continuing realization that it is essential in the interests of newer and more efficient ideas to use any existing plan only after checking every essential detail to ascertain the degree to which it should be modified for use in the next hospital.

THE CONCEPT OF TOTAL PROJECT MANAGEMENT

A comparatively new approach in construction which has made considerable advance in recent years has been the concept of 'total project management' or 'managed contracts,' to use two common terms.

Under the present system the owner deals with an architect, structural, electrical and mechanical engineers, a contractor and frequently a general consultant and often specialized consultants. The architect may have some

4 Ing. Jan Sliwa, 'The Oxford Method of System Building,' *World Hospitals*, vi, 3, July 1970, p. 161

jurisdiction over the engineers, but does not manage the contractor. Jurisdictional disputes may arise, responsibility on some points may be indefinite and, most seriously, time may be lost while cost escalation goes on and the most carefully calculated critical path or timing schedule is rendered futile.

In the managed contract one individual controls all the other parties. The project manager may be the contractor, the architect, the engineers, a special project management company or the owner himself. The main point is that there is one person who schedules the work of everybody else, co-ordinates the program and is more likely to complete the program on time within the budget. The project manager is directly responsible to the owner. The manager is frequently termed a 'turn-key' operator; in other words, he provides a complete service. Many large contractors in the United States work on this basis alone.

The managed contract method is being used increasingly in the hospital field. Hospital projects, because of their complexity, tend to drag on for months and estimates of cost quickly become obsolete. As I write, my consulting firm is working on a hospital project with a large turn-key contractor. The project is being funded by public subscription which is lamentably slow in reaching its goal. The turn-key contractor is on the point of borrowing the millions of dollars necessary to finish the project immediately; he is convinced that the heavy interest charges would be more than offset by escalating construction costs (if the project is delayed further) and the revenue from the earlier use of the hospital.

The concept is not without its critics. To maintain the estimated construction cost (possibly guaranteed, barring acts of God and of union leaders) the turn-key contractor may resist any change in plans. This can be a serious factor in hospitals where busy doctors are often late submitting what may be excellent ideas, but usually change orders can be negotiated. There is also always the possibility, when the architect is on the staff of the project manager or turn-key operator, that he may not be experienced in hospital design, or his experience may be dated. An architect once explained a hopelessly obsolete design to me by saying: 'I have done it this way for 35 years and I am not going to change now.' This enlightening conversation took place in the mid-sixties; the architect's illustration for the facility under discussion was dated 1929.

Also, where a construction figure is guaranteed there is a natural tendency under the stress of competition to make the figure as low as possible. With unforeseen increases in the cost of some items, there would be a natural tendency to effect compensatory economies in other items. The owners must check the specifications with great care to make sure they are adequately detailed. As construction proceeds the owners must make sure that continuing checks are made by someone well informed on the nature and quality of materials and equipment specified. Studies of some finished programs have indicated that the building committee seems to have given more attention to haggling over price than to the adequacy and quality of what was supplied. In the long run, of course, the possibility of poor planning and of shoddy construction to keep within the price must be largely self-limiting, for such policies soon give the firm which pursues them a bad reputation. But this is a principle that is harder to apply to hospital construction than to other less complex types of building.

7

Patterns of hospital care

In previous chapters we have seen how medical technology, improved standards and regulations, better qualifications of personnel at all levels, the removal of economic barriers through hospital and medical insurance, improved hospital design, and other factors have combined to transform the hospital from a charitable repository for indigents into a modern community medical centre. However, at the same time, parochial competition among some hospitals, the orientation of medical science toward acute episodic care and, most important of all, a general reluctance in society to recognize and provide for the needs of certain long-term patients have helped to create a 'non-system' of hospital and health care. In some cases there has been needless duplication and in others various health needs have been ignored almost completely.

SPECIALIZED HOSPITALS

For many years there have been specialty institutions – for the mentally ill, for the tuberculous, and for chronic and convalescent patients. Over the decades the relative number of specialized institutions for active treatment would seem to have decreased.

From the turn of the century until the first world war, hospitals were established in London, New York, Chicago and other metropolitan centres for the specific treatment of maternity, otolaryngology, ophthalmology, herniotomies, tropical diseases, neurology, heart disease, communicable diseases, urology, orthopaedics and other problems. Maternity hospitals, many of which were and are operated by the Salvation Army, became widespread in Canada. Most of the early specialty hospitals have become affiliated or absorbed into general hospitals. For instance the old Orthopaedic Hospital on Bloor Street West in Toronto (where the University Theatre now stands) which was directed by Dr B.E. Mackenzie and later by Dr Stewart Wright, was absorbed in the twenties into the renamed Toronto East General and Orthopaedic Hospital. (Dr Mackenzie had a large orthopaedic practice and was not liked by the teaching orthopods. Such was his natural flair for teaching that when he set up his own unofficial clinic demonstration on Saturday mornings, senior students in large numbers cut regular classes to go up to Bloor Street to hear him.)

Communicable-disease hospitals (usually municipally operated) and the federal government's quarantine hospitals became unnecessary as modern medicine brought communicable diseases under control; 'isolation by technique' became the practice in general hospitals. Many specialists, particularly otolaryngologists, moreover did not relish the separation from the general practitioners and other specialists that 'specialty' hospitals enforced. Some specialties like cardiology, orthopaedics and urology are better located in general hospitals. Although de Lee and other leading obstetricians thundered their insistence before the first world war that maternity patients be in a totally separate building, the improvement in technique and later the discovery of sulfa drugs and antibiotics made such separation unnecessary. If organisms continue to develop resistance to antibiotics we may, however, have to reverse our thinking.

Some specialty hospitals continue to thrive because they have organized excellent research as well as treatment efforts and maintained (or developed) public and medical support. The Montreal Neurological Hospital (affiliated with the Royal Victoria Hospital from 1934 until 1963) and the various cancer institutes with specialized, experienced staff (and the latest equipment) are good examples.

Another active treatment specialty hospital that is not being absorbed or discontinued is the children's hospital. There seems to be two reasons. First, it is, in most cases, really a general hospital for young people only. Second, the public is particularly sympathetic and responsive to financial appeals toward the sick child.

Canada has been fortunate in the development of an extraordinary number of good children's hospitals across the country. The Hospital for Sick Children in Toronto, which at present has more than 800 beds, dates from 1875 and for many years has been one of the leading research and postgraduate centres on the continent. For some years this hospital provided virtually the only paediatric beds in Toronto as a result of the widespread influence of John Ross Robertson, long-time chairman of the hospital's board. He persuaded local political leaders to establish civic regulations stipulating cutbacks in municipal financing to any hospital (other than his own) which operated a paediatric ward. In this way Toronto became unique among North American cities in having a single, very large children's hospital and minimal paediatric facilities in other hospitals.

The other Canadian general paediatric hospitals include the Montreal Children's Hospital, an institution with approximately 350 beds and an extensive building program now under way, which dates from 1904 and has a long history of brilliant achievement in teaching and research. L'Hôpital Ste Justine of Montreal was built in 1907. Under the enthusiastic leadership of Mme L. de G. Beaubien it moved in the late fifties into a modern new building, providing more than 800 beds for children and 50 for maternity patients. The Children's Hospital of Halifax, founded in 1909, became the Izaac Walton Killam Hospital for Children in 1970, with the building of a brand-new hospital of 325 beds on an adjacent site. The Children's Hospital in Winnipeg, which dates from 1910, moved into a fine new building of about 230 beds near the Winnipeg General Hospital in the fifties. It was the first children's hospital in Canada to develop surgical day centres. The Alberta Children's Hospital in Calgary, with a rated capacity of 130 beds, was formerly the Junior Red Cross Hospital for Crippled Children. The Children's Hospital in Vancouver was established in 1923 and has a capacity of 86 beds. For a number of years it has had plans for a new children's teaching hospital with more than 300 beds adjacent to the Vancouver General Hospital. The many hurdles to be cleared before it can be built have been discouraging. (In all my years as a planning consultant I have never seen as fine an outline of proposed requirements as has been worked out by this hospital.) A recent addition to this imposing list of children's hospitals is the Dr Charles A. Janeway Child Health Centre in St John's, Newfoundland. A new 320-bed children's hospital in Ottawa, the Children's Hospital of Eastern Ontario, was well advanced in its planning in 1970.

(Mention of the Ste Justine Hospital for Children in Montreal leads me into a diversion – a short introduction to the driving force behind that hospital, Mme L. de G. Beaubien. She was born with an abhorrence of idleness; for almost forty years she was president of Ste Justine and – for all practical purposes – its administrator as well. Seldom a day passed that she wasn't to be found in its corridors and she contributed heavily to its finances from her own purse. Her forceful personality and social standing pried many concessions from Premier Maurice Duplessis and Mayor Camilien Houde. When the new 850-bed hospital was under construction in the fifties, I had the privilege of being associated with her for several years. In addition to all her other attributes, she possessed an infallible sense of publicity. When it was time to break ground – or, rather, rock – she arranged a blast that alerted all of Montreal that the new Ste Justine's was underway. It was the first hospital in Canada to have a bombproof basement shelter and that was well publicised. When part of the roof was to be kept clear to permit a helicopter ambulance to land she said, 'Make space for three.' Then, with photographers and municipal officials standing by, three helicopters slowly descended on to the roof.

(At the time Ste Justine was the costliest hospital erected in Canada. Mme Beaubien's comment was typical: 'Costliest? It must be the *best* – anywhere.' She and her enthusiastic aide, Sister Noemi de Montfort, made an incomparable team. As the passing years took their toll, making her way around her beloved project became more difficult: the contractor presented her with her personal electric golf cart. She was named an honorary fellow of the American College of Hospital Administrators for her outstanding contributions.)

Specialized paediatric hospitals – for example, crippled children's centres and psychiatric hospitals – have also proliferated.

The outstanding care received in children's hospitals is reflected in the fact that all of the general and most of the specialized paediatric institutions have been accredited by the Canadian Council on Hospital Accreditation.

CONVALESCENT AND EXTENDED-CARE HOSPITALS

One of the greatest gaps in the health-care system of Canada has been the perpetual insufficiency of beds, services and other facilities specifically designed for convalescent and chronically ill patients. Medical science has been predominantly oriented to acute episodic care; physicians have concentrated their efforts on diagnosis and treatment of such diseases. Many procedures requiring the skill of a physician are not so prominent in the treatment and care of convalescents and the chronically ill. To be sure, some chronic ailments periodically require the full medical resources of the acute-care hospital but generally these conditions can be treated adequately with less direct medical supervision.

Unfortunately not enough qualified physicians have shown enough interest to provide adequately for even the limited medical needs of extended-care patients. This neglect has been reflected in the community by the low priority traditionally given to the financing of facilities and services for those needing prolonged care. Yet the need for long-term care has dramatically increased during this century as a result of advances in medical science and public health measures which have greatly altered disease patterns and increased the average life expectancy.

Most convalescent and chronically ill patients have been and are treated in the home. However, as the years have passed, our homes have generally become smaller as have our families; few of us can afford live-in domestic help – even if such gems were available. In all, the conditions which previously made home care practical have almost disappeared.

Chronic and convalescent patients requiring intensive medical care usually have been treated in the general hospital. However, in conformity with hospital trends toward specialization, some chronic disease and convalescent hospitals have been established as separate institutions. Because most extended-care patients have less need for the expensive facilities such as oxygen, air climatization, sophisticated radiological equipment, diagnostic laboratories, operating rooms and so on, there is a reluctance to put such patients in the acute general hospital. In addition the chronically ill have their own special needs for more privacy and special rehabilitative and recreational facilities.

The convalescent or chronic unit operated as a wing of a general hospital has always been the least expensive to operate. This relationship, which originated in France, was followed in London, Chicago and elsewhere. It provided minimal difficulties in transferring and transporting patients and facilitated some continuity of care.

However, many long-term patients prefer to be away from the urban noise and pollution and seek relative tranquillity, sunshine and fresh air. For this reason and because the required recreational, rehabilitative and other facilities were generally similar, many chronic and convalescent hospitals are modelled after tuberculosis sanatoria. The buildings are often of two-storey construction situated at some distance from the city centre, containing many private rooms, sitting rooms and solaria and surrounded by grounds for ambulatory patients.

Hillcrest Convalescent Hospital in Toronto, built in 1886, is the oldest such institution in Canada. Several chronic-care hospitals in Quebec date from the same period. By the 1920s there were more than fifty institutions providing some 2,500 chronic and convalescent care beds. Many were privately owned and provided little more than food and shelter and offered practically no nursing service. Even for the voluntary hospitals there was no generally accepted standard concerning what types of patients should be admitted. Many institutions drastically limited their clientele, accepting patients who required no dressings or special diets. In a few cases bedridden patients were not admitted. Some of these institutions had no laboratory facilities, no medical supervision, no physiotherapy nor hydrotherapy, no occupational nor recreational therapy, no dietitian, no orderly service, and were not deserving, in fact, of the name hospital.

There were a few institutions which did provide superior treatment and care, mostly in Montreal and Toronto. The Deer Lodge Veterans' Hospital in Winnipeg was also considered to have some of the finest and best equipped extended care facilities on the continent. I have enjoyed a most rewarding experience over a great many years as a trustee of St John's Convalescent Hospital in Toronto.[1] Originated by Anglican Sisters with a lay board, it is an institution which provides a very high quality of care.

Available statistics are somewhat misleading in that many institutions provided less than hospital standard service but by 1942 there were some 4,400 beds in 31 voluntary convalescent chronic and domiciliary care 'hospitals.' There were also some 136 private hospitals and nursing homes giving long-term care. In 1948, at the commencement of the national health grant program, voluntary chronic and convalescent hospitals had a combined rated bed capacity of approximately 3,700. In 1958 this figure had grown to more than 10,500. In 1969 some 116 chronic, rehabilitative and convalescent hospitals contained more than 15,500 beds.

Although per diem costs were generally 30 to 50 percent lower in convalescent-care hospitals, the long-term nature of the diseases made it financially impossible for many patients in the twenties and thirties to receive the treatment they needed. The Blue Cross hospital insurance plans did little to relieve the situation as coverage per year was generally limited to three weeks or a month. The inability of many persons to pay for prolonged care further aggravated the shortage of extended-care facilities. It was for this reason that the federal government gave higher grants for the construction of convalescent and chronic-care hospitals than for other institutions under the national health grants program. More beds in all hospitals – but especially in long-term institutions – were necessary before hospital insurance could be introduced.

The Hospital Insurance and Diagnostic Services Act of 1957 provided for coverage of chronic and convalescent hospital care at the discretion of

---

1 In recognition of his services, the new addition at St John's, expected to be completed in 1974, is to be named the G. Harvey Agnew Wing.

each province. All provincial governments moved rapidly to take advantage of this option.

MENTAL HOSPITALS AND INSTITUTIONS

Somewhere in the dark distant origins of civilization our ancestors were afflicted with a fear-hate complex about mental illness and we have only started to work our way out of it. Even in the twentieth century mental illness has been regarded by many as the invasion of the soul by devils and demons. Physicians and rational men have been convinced for centuries that there are no supernatural forces at work in the mentally sick but in no area of human endeavor have superstition and prejudice taken so long to overcome.

Today, early in the eighth decade of the twentieth century, many Canadians still attach a stigma to mental illness and attempt to disguise, ignore or deny its existence.

Until the nineteenth century the usual methods of 'treating' mental illness were starvation, bleeding, purging, beatings, exorcism and the more severe measures of torture and burning. By the middle of the last century society had progressed to the point of simply 'putting away' or 'committing' the mentally ill where necessary, often in institutions that were not considered fit for the common criminal. New enlightenment occasionally opened a few windows through the efforts of such outstanding psychiatrists as Dorothea Dix in the United States, who had the shackles removed from patients in various state asylums (and who was instrumental in having the Nova Scotia Hospital built in 1858). In Canada, Dr Joseph Workman of Toronto, Dr R.M. Bucke of London, Ontario, Dr C.K. Clarke and, later, Dr C.M. Hincks of Toronto led the way in revolutionizing medical attitudes about illness. By the late 1920s, mental illness was receiving close scrutiny and mental hospitals, most of which were built as custodial institutions, were offering an increasing scope and intensity of treatment.

Almost all severe psychiatric illnesses, as well as much retardation and senility, were treated in provincially owned and operated institutions,[2] many of which were designed by prison architects and contained anywhere from 400 to 600 beds. No reliable national statistics are available before 1929; at that time there were 26,862 beds in forty-two mental hospitals. That is, *there were almost as many patients in mental institutions as in all*

---

2 Except in Nova Scotia, where 'county homes' have long been municipally owned, and in Quebec, where religious orders have traditionally run the mental hospitals. Only during the sixties have lay members assumed greater direction of these latter hospitals.

the public general hospitals. This situation continued unabated until the 1960s when advances in drug therapy and improved out-patient and home-care services permitted a higher rate of early discharges.

The mental hospitals in the twenties were built to last forever. The windows were barred and the doors bolted. Unfortunately, it was not generally appreciated, at least on a conscious level, that people tend to live up to the roles expected of them – in this case to be violent and often dangerous. Such an environment was not therapeutic, especially for the considerable majority of inmates who were non-violent. The senile and mentally retarded made up a large proportion of the patients and suffered the same lack of privacy and dignity afforded to the psychiatrically ill. Large dormitories provided most of the sleeping accommodation so that patients were under the immediate supervision of the ward attendant at all times. Recreational and social activities were minimal. Overcrowding was prevalent and dehumanizing. Mental hospitals were designed so that patients were normally crowded and still the administrators squeezed in even more so that the beds in use always exceeded the rated capacity.

Other problems included a perpetual shortage of qualified staff; inadequate provision of medical care for physical ailments due to the usual semi-isolation of mental hospitals; and failure to diagnose psychiatric illnesses at an early stage which resulted in prolonged regression for many patients. Problems of overcrowding, as a result of an accumulation of chronically ill or senile patients having little or no need for psychiatric treatment, were relieved only in Nova Scotia, where a system of county homes was set up in 1878 for the chronically ill and senile.

The greatest problem – and causal factor of all of others to some extent – was the attitude of the public and politicians who refused to provide adequate financial support for mental hospitals.

The public regarded mental illness for the most part as a disgrace. The popular reaction was rejection of the mental patient, often isolating him to a far away institution and then denying more than minimal responsibility for his plight.

Community treatment was mostly unavailable. It was the day of the 'snake pit' mental hospitals – bars, locks, restraints, 'herding' and all the rest ...

Patients were admitted by legal process and retained in locked wards. Because of understaffing and overcrowding, the emphasis was on custody rather than therapy. Patients and their relatives used the hospital only as a last resort. Mental illness evoked feelings of shame and hopelessness in the families of the mentally ill; many were encouraged to forget the patient following his admission.[3]

3 Department of National Health and Welfare, *National Health Grants 1948–1961*, p. 134

There were, of course many outstanding psychiatrists dedicated to improving methods and facilities for treatment. Dr J.J. MacNeill, superintendent at North Battleford for many years and later Saskatchewan commissioner of mental services; Dr A.L. Crease of British Columbia; Dr B.T. McGhie of Ontario; Dr A.E. Moll of Quebec, Dr D.G. McKerracher of Saskatchewan; Dr Charles Roberts, originally from St John's, Newfoundland, were among the pioneers.

In 1930 Ontario introduced a system of mental health clinics, encouraging community participation through subsidies. In this effort to provide services to those unable to pay and to make psychiatric services more widely available, clinics were established in mental hospitals, public hospitals and under separate auspices. Somewhat later Nova Scotia adopted this concept and opened a community mental health clinic in each of nine regions.

In Montreal such progressive measures as the 'open door,' day-and-night hospitals (first in 1946 at the Allan Memorial Institute of the Royal Victoria Hospital in Montreal) and admissions wards were introduced and began to spread after the second world war.

The first coverage of psychiatric treatment by health insurance plans was instituted in Saskatchewan under the Hospital Insurance Act in 1947. At first the coverage was limited to treatment received in general hospitals but was extended to mental hospitals in 1948. Nova Scotia followed in 1949, and by 1970 insurance coverage was available in all provinces.

Another landmark was the construction of small mental hospitals of 300 beds or fewer to serve a small region. These institutions have served their surrounding communities exclusively; they have maintained all the advantages of mental health clinics and in addition have provided a much greater range of diagnostic and treatment services. Many of these regional mental hospitals, a growing few of the larger and older ones, together with the psychiatric units in public general hospitals, are operated by local administrative authorities. Decentralization of provincial control and greater community participation in provision of services for the mentally ill is the stated policy of several provinces. As an illustration, the Lakeshore Psychiatric Hospital in Etobicoke (formerly New Toronto) in the late sixties was managed by a lay board with considerable authority within the financial restrictions and regulations defined by the provincial department of health. This decentralization has done a great deal to bring the hospital and the community closer together. Progress in this area, however, continues to be slow.

In Saskatchewan in 1944 psychiatric nursing courses were introduced for non-RN's and have helped to improve the qualification of staff. Today the four western provinces have nine schools offering two-year psychiatric nursing diploma courses. In addition there are continuing education courses in psychiatry for RN's across the country. Psychologists, occupational therapists and psychiatric social workers are also slowly being accepted as part of the mental health team in psychiatric hospitals. In-service education, a rarity only fifteen years ago, has now become commonplace in mental hospitals. A gradual increase in psychiatric training in medical schools has attracted more and better qualified doctors into psychiatry. All of these developments have improved staff qualifications and have alleviated somewhat the shortage of psychiatrists.

In treatment the development which has had the greatest effect has been chemotherapy. In the early fifties the pharmaceutical houses began introducing such drugs as the phenothiazine derivatives and the diphenylethanes which have stabilized the conditions of many mentally ill persons, often for prolonged periods. Thus even though chronic-care psychiatric and mentally retarded patients have increased considerably in number (largely owing to a longer life span) discharges of newly diagnosed patients have reached an all-time high. In addition out-patient clinics, day and/or night hospitals and home-care services have proven adequate for an increasing number of patients. By 1966 the total number of patients in mental institutions and especially psychiatric hospitals had begun to drop, not only in terms relative to the population but in absolute figures. In the Saskatchewan Hospital at Weyburn the patient census decreased by 50 percent between 1963 and 1965. The trend has continued and accelerated. In 1970 there were approximately 60,000 beds in mental hospitals, a reduction of about 15 percent since 1966.

With a few exceptions the new mental hospitals built since 1920 have been smaller – only occasionally of more than 400 beds – and generally more specialized. With increasing frequency, epileptics, the mentally retarded, senile patients, short-term and chronically ill psychiatric patients have been segregated in separate facilities. Similarly children have been treated in separate units and often in separate hospitals.

PSYCHIATRIC UNITS IN GENERAL HOSPITALS

The establishment of psychiatric units as part of public general hospitals has been advocated for many decades in Canada, at first with limited success. In the 1920s and 1930s little attention was paid to the care of psychiatric patients. 'Psychosomatic medicine' was a term just coming into the vocabulary of the profession. Psychoses were considered as a subject quite apart from internal medicine and were so taught to us as students. Among my own teachers, only Dr William Goldie and Dr George F. Young considered psychiatric factors in medical conditions. The former advised us to buy tie pins, then an essential part of male accoutrement, in the form of a question mark. The question symbolically posed, he said, should be a guide throughout our professional lives. Dr Young had begun as a general practitioner and was quickly becoming regarded as one of Toronto's leading medical consultants, largely because he considered the whole patient and gave nearly as much thought to his social and financial background as to his physical condition.

Few hospitals of the time had the psychiatric wards so common today. One teaching hospital in Toronto – the Toronto General Hospital – had a psychiatric unit located in the superintendent's residence as early as 1906. This ward was incorporated into the hospital when it moved from the east end of Toronto to its present site in 1912. (I speculate, but it may have been built because the superintendent, Dr C.K. Clarke, was a leading psychiatrist. It may also have been because Dr Sigmund S. Goldwater, then superintendent of Mount Sinai Hospital in New York City and for many years America's leading hospital planning consultant, was consultant on the planning of this new hospital. Unfortunately, once built, the new unit was not used to provide the psychiatric care for which it was planned.)

Although psychiatric wards in general hospitals did not become common until after the second world war, it should be noted that the Pennsylvania Hospital in Philadelphia, of which Benjamin Franklin was one of the founders, has had a psychiatric ward from the beginning. General hospitals were not keen on admitting psychiatric patients and did so only under restrictions. Some hospitals had a special room, frequently in the basement, where cases of delirium tremens and other mentally disturbed patients were confined. As in regular mental hospitals, the locked door, the peephole and the barred windows were enough to seriously agitate any confused individual. Private patients were placed in a single room, often with the obligation to have special nurses or attendants around the clock. There were no tranquilizers as such and general sedation was used to settle a disturbed person. If the patient was noisy and violently disturbed, a lumbar puncture was done to relieve cerebrospinal pressure, a risky and even dangerous procedure under the circumstances.

Few general hospitals had a staff psychiatrist; in fact, there were few psychiatrists in private practice. Nearly all were on the staff of mental hospitals. Hence few were available in cities without such an institution. In larger centres, one of the staff of a nearby mental hospital would be called in when needed; more frequently the patient was transferred to the mental hospital without delay. If the distance was great these patients were transferred by rail, frequently under police guard. Such was the situation in northern Ontario where disturbed patients had to be transported long distances to southern Ontario institutions. In some cases Winnipeg and other Manitoba centres would have been closer but Manitoba was not about to accommodate mental patients from northern Ontario as a matter of routine.

So far has the pendulum swung in recent years that many hospitals of only 150 to 200 beds have special psychiatric units. In Quebec, indeed, the province may withhold building funds if the added accommodation does not make provision for psychiatric treatment. (Very small hospitals are usually excused from this provision.)

But, I hasten to add, not all our large and medium-sized hospitals provide psychiatric wards. Some of our larger hospitals believe that the type of mild psychotic whom they should admit, either with or without a concomitant physical ailment, should be treated as any other patient, including admission to a multi-bed room. If symptoms or mental reactions develop which would be disturbing or dangerous to others, tranquilizers or other drugs are used to control the situation, perhaps with transfer of the patient to a single room. The disadvantage of this arrangement is that it is not always possible to anticipate or readily control the reactions of some patients. Also, unless all of the rooms where such patients might be housed are equipped with special window safeguards, tamper-proof light switches, alarm bells on emergency exits and so on, the danger of suicide is much greater. Nervous non-psychotic patients are often perturbed if they must share a room, or even be on the same corridor, with certain wandering types of mental patients.

More encouragement is given today to the family practitioner to follow up his psychiatric patients in the general hospital. While many psychiatric patient units are closed to other than certified psychiatrists and associated psychologists, in others the psychiatrists in charge encourage the family physician to generally direct the care of the patient under the guidance and supervision of the psychiatrist. This is good medicine. The patients tend to have more confidence in the doctor whom they know than in a stranger; the family doctor is better acquanted with the individual and his social background; and, still, the wisdom of the psychiatrist is there to ensure the best care for the patient.

THE CANADIAN MENTAL HEALTH ASSOCIATION

Dr Clarence M. Hincks of Toronto was the driving force behind the establishment of the Committee on Mental Health in 1918. This federation of provincial organizations became the Canadian Council of Mental Hygiene in 1939 and the Canadian Mental Health Association in 1950.

With the assistance of Dr C.K. Clarke and Marjorie Keyes of Toronto and Dr C.F. Martin and Dr C.K. Russell of Montreal, the committee (association) conducted surveys, petitioned governments and helped to improve the attitude of the public and politicians toward mental illness. It has sponsored research and financed volunteer services and White Cross centres.

Dr J.D. Griffin succeeded Dr Hincks as executive director in the early 1950s.

TUBERCULOSIS HOSPITALS

Towards the end of the nineteenth century tuberculosis terrorized the citizens of this country. With a death rate approaching 200 per 100,000, the 'white plague' was the No. 1 killer in Canada. For many years people believed that the disease was hereditary and incurable and reacted to a positive diagnosis as they would to a death sentence.

In 1882 the German dentist, Robert Koch, isolated the tubercle bacillus and proved tuberculosis to be infectious. The sequential implication that TB was controllable and preventable was not universally recognized at first. But by the turn of the century voluntary agencies such as the Canadian Tuberculosis Association and the National Sanatorium Association had initiated fund-raising campaigns to build hospitals for the tuberculous. The first was constructed on a hill overlooking Lake Muskoka near Gravenhurst, Ontario, in 1896. Others followed in such places as Kentville, Nova Scotia (1904), Toronto (1904), Lac Edouard, Quebec (1904), Hamilton (1906), Tranquille, British Columbia (1907), Ste Agathe des Monts and surrounding communities in the Laurentians (from 1908), Ninette, Manitoba (1910) and London, Ontario (1910).

These first sanatoria were erected well out in the country, far from city noises and other disturbances, and with a pleasant view and clean air. Many patients spent as long as two years confined in them and boredom was a perpetual problem, usually alleviated in those early days only by a sparsely stocked library. Visitors were discouraged by the inaccessibility of most tuberculosis hospitals. Bed capacity was determined by a ratio of one bed to each patient death per year in those days of sunshine, overfeeding and freezing.

Unfortunately most diagnoses of consumption were made in the office of a physician only when symptoms had become visible and so obvious that the patient himself usually correctly feared the worst. By that time, of course, treatment had been too long delayed and death almost invariably resulted.

To help facilitate earlier diagnosis clinics were established, the first in 1909 at the Royal Edward Institute in Montreal. These were sponsored initially by voluntary associations (or occasionally by municipal authorities); an increasing share of the financial burden of these and other public health measures to detect and prevent TB has however been assumed by government agencies over the years.

Informing and educating the public was crucial. The effectiveness of sanatorium care, limited in any case, was severely reduced by late detection and reluctance of patients to be admitted. The voluntary associations accepted responsibility for much of the education and publicity required to win massive public support and co-operation. 'Early discovery aids early recovery' was a well-used publicity slogan. Eventually, when financial barriers had been greatly reduced or eliminated, provinces legislated compulsory admission to sanatoria for all TB victims.

By 1921 the death rate for tuberculosis had fallen markedly to 87.7 per 100,000. The growing sophistication of X-ray equipment which permitted earlier diagnosis and the segregation of patients were probably the most important factors in this decline. But remarkable as these advances were, even greater inroads in eliminating the disease have been made since that time.

During the twenties and thirties the emphasis continued on adequate sanatoria facilities and improvement of means of diagnosis. The tuberculin test came into use as a preliminary means of diagnosis. The BCG (bacillus calmetta guerin) vaccine, which provided about 80 percent immunity, was administered to a growing number of medical and nursing personnel, children, and others who ran high risks of exposure. L'Hôpital Marie Enfant in Montreal was conceived in mid-1930s as a provincial vaccination centre for infants and small children and for many years a widespread BCG program was conducted in Quebec.

Thoracic surgery was used extensively, the Weston Sanatorium in Toronto being the first to install surgical facilities of its own in 1930.

It was during this period that the provincial governments assumed much greater responsibilities for the operation and maintenance of treatment facilities. In so many cases patients simply could not afford the prolonged treatment and were forced to discontinue their programs or face bankruptcy. In 1929 Saskatchewan began paying the entire treatment costs of all TB patients. On that occasion the Saskatchewan Anti-Tuberculosis

League, formed in 1911, became a semi-public agency with provincial and municipal representatives on its board of directors. Alberta followed Saskatchewan's example in 1933 and today all provinces pay the entire cost of tuberculosis treatment (except in a few cases where the patient is expected to pay a nominal amount if he can afford it).

For many years organized X-ray surveys were restricted to students of medicine and nursing and a few high incidence communities. During the second world war the first massive survey originated when all personnel recruited to and discharged from the armed services received chest X-rays. By 1950, with considerable aid from the national health grants program, mass surveys were extended to all school children and hospital admission X-rays became routine. These same federal government funds, totalling about $4 million annually, were used to improve sanatoria services substantially.

The last quarter century can justly be called the era of chemotherapy. Drugs such as streptomycin, isoniazed, para-aminosalicylic acid and others have worked miracles in reducing not only the death rate but the incidence of TB. From a peak year (in absolute figures) of approximately 6.25 million treatment days in 1953 provided at a cost of $32 million, public sanatoria spent less than $27 million on just more than a million treatment days in 1969. There are, in fact, a host of statistics demonstrating the potential elimination of tuberculosis. Sanatoria are closing each year; occupancy is at an all-time low (65 percent in 1969 as opposed to 93 percent in 1953) despite the fact that rated bed capacities are declining everywhere; the mortality rate is less than three per 100,000 and, most important, the incidence of reported new cases is steadily declining (approximately 22 per 100,000 in 1969 as against 125.3 per 100,000 in 1944).

Due to the relatively high incidence of TB among physicians and medical students, many doctors became interested in returning to care for tuberculosis patients following their own recovery. It was the writer's privilege to enjoy the acquaintance and friendship of many outstanding 'ex-lungers' and other leaders in the tuberculosis field. Names such as Drs J.H. Holbrook of Hamilton, D.A. Steward of Ninette, Manitoba, R.G. Ferguson of Fort San, Fort Qu'Appelle, Saskatchewan, J.A. Couillard of Lac Edouard, Quebec, H.A. Farris of Saint John, New Brunswick, Baker of Calgary, W.J. Dobbie, J.H. Elliott and G.C. Brink of Toronto and G.J. Wherrett of Ottawa, come immediately to mind. The relentless efforts of these determined physicians and their colleagues have set the stage for the final drive to eliminate tuberculosis in Canada.

Treatment in General Hospitals

Before the wonder drugs came into the picture beginning in the late forties, the average length of stay in sanatoria was approximately eighteen months. The long-term and infectious nature of the disease as well as the specialized treatment involved dictated that most patients be isolated in sanatoria.

By the late forties, these hospitals were usually equipped with a large auditorium or meeting hall for movies, other entertainment and religious services, beauty and barber shops, a library, canteen and facilities for occupational therapy and vocational training. Naturally, some of these facilities were not readily available in many general hospitals.

Today the average stay has been reduced to two months and the infectious stage rarely lasts more than a couple of weeks. Medical reasons for continued isolation in sanatoria have been largely eradicated.

In recent years difficulty has risen in maintaining competent medical staff in sanatoria due to lack of competitive remuneration and a belief among many medical students that a career in tuberculosis treatment does not hold a satisfying future. By integrating tuberculosis patients into special infectious or respiratory disease wards of the general hospital they would come under the continuous care and supervision of expert internists.

However, there are a variety of other factors involved in transferring TB victims to general hospital, not the least of which is cost. General hospital beds have always been much more expensive to maintain than have sanatoria beds. However, as occupancy rates fall, as they have for some time in tuberculosis hospitals, the cost per patient per day rises. The conversion of sanatoria beds to serve convalescing patients or the chronically ill has been made difficult by the location of the institutions, their structure, and often their age. Where conversion has been possible occupancy rates have risen and great savings have been effected.

The Canadian Tuberculosis Association

Since its founding in 1900 the Canadian Tuberculosis Association has sprouted some 200 local branches as well as the ten provincial and one territorial (Yukon) associations. Originally conceived as to build and operate sanatoria, the voluntary organization's functions were extended to include sponsorship of a variety of measures to promote, in co-operation with provincial and local health departments, the early detection and prevention of TB. The CTA has also become actively involved in rehabilitation and, more recently, research programs.

The traditional method of fund raising began in Canada in 1908 when the

Toronto and Hamilton associations sold Christmas seals. By 1927 the Christmas seal campaign had become the offical means for all branches of the CTA to raise money. In 1970 more than one million Canadians donated more than $3 million to combat TB and other chest illnesses.

The CTA became the Canadian Tuberculosis and Respiratory Disease Association in 1968, reflecting an increasing concern with other respiratory ailments but 'until complete eradication has been attained, that is, until the disease (TB) has disappeared and all forms of action except surveillance can be abandoned, the CTRDA will continue to concentrate a large part of its efforts on the control of tuberculosis.'[4]

THE GENERAL HOSPITAL

For generations the general hospitals in Canada have looked after the severely ill who came within the restricted acute-care category. The general hospitals were not very interested in patients needing other types of care, especially if they were more troublesome to handle, or suffered from conditions that lacked popular appeal, did not show quick results, or were difficult to finance. If the general hospital continued to care for the chronically ill or the convalescent who had nobody at home, it was only because they could not be sent away elsewhere. Even then there were complaints that these patients took up beds badly needed for others. Furthermore, when patients were discharged the general hospital cared little about what happened to them and what follow-up existed was left entirely to their personal physician if they had one.

Only very gradually have we begun to look at the patient as a whole and done something about carrying him through – not only his acute illness or accident – until his rehabilitation is complete or at least maximized.

At the same time that this determination to provide more comprehensive care in, or in conjunction with, the general hospital was rising, the increasing costs of various types of specialized equipment and intensive care, as well as the shortage of qualified medical and nursing personnel, dictated a more efficient utilization of resources.

For years in the big general wards nurses put the seriously ill patients close to the nurses' desk. The less seriously ill were located in the more remote areas of the unit, possibly near the sun porch, if one existed. The chronically ill were occasionally put in the older building when a new one

4 C.W.L. Jeanes and Carla Gilders, *Canadian Journal of Public Health*, March 1970, p. 153

went up. Together with the post-anaesthetic room, this was the extent of segregation of in-patients by severity of illness.

Beginning in the 1950s a few hospitals espoused a concept called 'progressive patient care' in which patients were shifted from one type of accommodation to another as the severity of their condition changed while in hospital. Previously, patients were grouped almost exclusively by type of illness (for example, medical, surgical, paediatric); the new arrangement, while less convenient for the medical specialists in some cases, promised greater overall efficiency.

However, many patients and hospital personnel have adamantly opposed a full program of intensive patient care on the legitimate grounds that it disrupts the continuity of patient care. To have a patient admitted to a self-care unit while tests are done, transferred to surgery, then intensive care, followed by acute care, convalescent care and finally a home-care program all within two or three weeks means that his doctors and nurses will be changing constantly. He is likely to be treated more as a body passing through than as a person.

What we have observed over the past ten years has been an attempt by hospitals to balance effective continuity of care and 'progressive patient care,' selecting from the latter concept only those features which have been practical and of definite benefit to the patient. The intensive care unit (ICU) and the home-care program have been the most widely adopted facets of progressive patient care.

The Intensive Care Unit
The number of beds in an intensive care unit can vary considerably. Unless there are at least four to six beds it hardly can warrant the near-continual presence of physicians. When it is larger than sixteen to twenty beds, it has sometimes proven difficult to maintain the tempo of care required. However, some units have been larger and categorization is frequently more loosely done in these cases. Naturally the intensity and quality of care in ICUs has varied among hospitals depending on staff training and equipment.

The need for intensive care units has been questionable if the hospital has had fewer than 150 beds and some have placed the minimal size even higher. In smaller hospitals it has been as effective and more economical to have a few severely ill patients near the nursing station given a special staffing ratio. In some instances the end of a nursing unit has been set aside for intensive care. These arrangements have permitted flexibility in use.

In 1970 there were some twenty-one hundred intensive care beds in more than 250 hospitals in Canada.

Home Care
Dr E.M. Bluestone of the Montefiore Hospital in New York City never tired of emphasizing that the best way to ensure that doctors do not keep chronic or convalescent patients unnecessarily long in active treatment beds and to generally avoid over-utilization of expensive hospital resources was to provide excellent alternatives. There have always been many patients requiring a level of care and treatment unavailable in the home but not so intense as provided in chronic care, convalescent and other extended-care units or institutions. Besides extensive out-patient services the most obvious alternative to over-utilization of hospital beds was organized home care.

Most doctors used to make house calls, of course, but unless the illness was not serious and of short duration, the physician simply could not spare the time personally to give the required treatment and care in the home. Local visiting nurse services have existed in Canada since the 1940s and on a national scale since 1897 and although the services given were of superior quality they were often not enough. What was needed was a physician-directed program which co-ordinated and integrated the services of the visiting nurses, with a broad range of hospital and other social services.

There were a few scattered home-care programs, providing organized and integrated services in the northeastern United States in the last century. In 1930 Chicago established an ambitious comprehensive medical care program which included home care but it wasn't until 1947 and the Montefiore Hospital home-care program that interest in such services became widespread.

The first hospital-based home-care program in Canada originated at the Reddy Memorial Hospital in Montreal in 1950. Faced with a shortage of general hospital beds, concerned about rising construction and operating costs and searching for methods to generate interest in general practice among interns, the hospital and the Victorian Order of Nurses set up a basic home-care service for carefully selected patients. Interns and nurses were assigned in accordance with the wishes of the patient's private physician or the chief of service (for public-ward patients). Co-operation was the key in this and all subsequent home-care programs – co-operation among the von, the home-care section and all other hospital departments and outside community social agencies. Crucially important was the co-operation and support of physicians.

With funds from the national health grants program, hospitals or community agencies in co-operation with hospitals began various programs during the fifties. Vernon, British Columbia, established a convalescent home nursing service in 1951 and was followed by the Winnipeg General Hospital and the pilot home-care program in Toronto in 1958. At the time of writing there were home-care programs in most major centres across the country.

So long as home-care services remained uninsured many physicians were reluctant to refer some of their hospital insured patients to them, especially those for whom the charges would be a financial burden. In 1964 the Ontario Hospital Services Commission began sponsoring an expanded Metropolitan Toronto home-care program.

Beside physicians and visiting nurses, home-care programs have come to employ a wide range of professional and technical personnel and facilities available to hospital patients. In order to supplement and facilitate the application of health measures, homemaker services, 'meals on wheels,' friendly visitors and other services have been made available. The cost of each program depends on the scope of the services available and the frequency with which they are employed. In the late 1960s, average costs were approximately $8 to $9 per diem. Although these costs were comparable to treatment (as opposed to accommodation plus treatment) costs in some extended-care institutions, the approach ensures a more efficient use of available resources by keeping the patient at home, rather than providing more institutional beds. The prime advantage of treating patients at home, however, is that they receive adequate care in a familiar environment which helps them to maintain their good spirits and independence. Home care must not be thought of as a substitute for active treatment hospital care, nor even for chronic or convalescent hospital care. It is rather an alternative method of health care which best satisfies the needs of certain patients, mostly elderly and chronically ill, whose condition and home environment meet various medical and social criteria.

Ambulatory Care
We have seen how the active treatment general hospital has greatly increased the scope of its services since 1920, by incorporating the functions of most of the active treatment specialty hospitals, by treating an increasing number of psychiatric and tuberculosis patients and by sponsor-

ing or participating in home-care programs. In many ways the most profound changes in the function of the general hospital have concerned the care of the ambulatory patient.

The hospital care of out-patients is by no means a new story. It is probably the oldest basis of treatment, for the priest-physicians who presided over the pagan temples of Egypt in the time of Imhotep 3,000 years before Christ apparently could treat the supplicant sufferers who were brought to them only on an out-patient basis. Nor should we overlook the Babylonian priests who presided over their temples and invoked miracles from the sun god Shamash on those who came to them.

But out-patient care has changed considerably over this half century. In the twenties and thirties the out-patient departments of the large urban city hospitals were heavily patronized. Hospitals like the Montreal General Hospital and the Toronto General Hospital had, and still have, unusually heavy demands, reminiscent of the services in London, Edinburgh and on the continent, or of the larger clinics in the United States. The out-patient clinics were basically for those who could not pay a private physician. In my own hospital in Toronto the registration fee was 10 cents – if the patient could afford it. (As I write I note in one of the hospital journals that the going rate in many of the larger American hospitals is $15 and more). Our out-patient doctors became exceedingly angry at patients who booked in wearing an expensive fur coat and sometimes with a good car waiting. For that lack of judgment by the patient there could have been a grain of truth in the rumor that the doctor giving his time gratis sometimes got a little personal satisfaction by including in the treatment some laxative notorious for its prolonged explosive effect.

We also had many patients who had little wrong with them but came repeatedly, possibly for something to do, possibly for the personal attention. Cartoonists in *Punch* frequently singled such out. Our ear, nose and throat service was headed by Dr Nathan McKinley, an ardent Queen's graduate. ('Ardent' may be a redundant adjective, for are there any Queen's men who are *not* ardent Queen's men, or women who are not even more so?) McKinley was a busy man with a fairly low boiling point and his favourite diagnosis for these patients, as recorded on the case card, was 'NADT' which, on interpretation, meant simply 'not a damn thing.'

The hospitals in smaller cities usually had only a few special clinics – tuberculosis once or twice a month and a VD clinic in some. Small hospitals usually had none; the doctors preferred to treat indigents in their own offices than spend time in a poorly patronized clinic. Low-income patients had more pride then and most did not hastily accept free service. In the

Prairie provinces, clinics, apart from special ones mentioned above, were few, even in the larger cities. Doctors were accustomed to carrying patients through bad crop years and preferred to take their chances on some degree of later payment.

With the depression years in the early thirties and the development of welfare relief measures, it became possible in some provinces for the doctors to see patients on relief in their own offices and receive varying amounts of payment from welfare funds. This reduced the pressure on the clinics in many hospitals although others did not notice much change. Many 'paying' patients were going to a local hospital on instruction from their private physician for X-ray, for laboratory work, or for physical therapy. They, however, went directly to the department designated and had no contact with the out-patient department or the emergency unit.

Non-Admitted Private Care by Appointment
Following the second world war the picture changed considerably. As medical progress advanced, more and more studies required for an exact diagnosis could be done only in hospital. The knowledge gained by 'inquiry, inspection, palpation and auscultation' had to be supplemented with increasing frequency by laboratory and radiological findings. This required more and more referral to the hospital. Moreover, the many minor procedures formerly done in the office or at home were done less and less in the office and almost never in the home. Nurses were in such short supply that few doctors had them any more in the office; a typist with a limited knowledge of simple office procedures became the doctor's only office assistant.

It was much simpler, a time saver and safer for the patient to have minor procedures such as removal of cysts or growths, setting of simple fractures, reapplying of casts and some of the less exacting endoscopy procedures done in the hospital – usually in emergency and often by scheduled appointment. In some cases senior staff physicians had offices in the hospital (usually a teaching one) or in an adjacent building where it was quite convenient to go to the out-patient department for tests and minor therapy.

This practice in the fifties and sixties became so widespread that, in many hospitals with an active emergency department, the limited space often made it difficult to proceed with appointments at the arranged times or to handle emergencies when they came in. During the sixties planners began to provide facilities for these non-admitted ambulatory patients adjacent to the emergency department but not interfering with the desirable 'readiness-to-serve' of that department. The privilege to treat patients on this ambulatory basis has been of course, a matter of decision by the proper committee of the medical staff. This ambulatory service has largely replaced the concept of low-cost out-patient clinics except in those larger metropolitan hospitals where there is still a demand for these services, to a large extent by new Canadians accustomed to such facilities.

For some years several provincial government insurance plans did not adequately cover out-patient services. As benefits have gradually and extensively been introduced to the ambulatory patient, this has helped to relieve pressure for more beds, promoted greater efficiency and generally encouraged a great expansion of out-patient facilities.

The Emergency Department
Traditionally this has been a service of all active treatment hospitals, irrespective of whether they also maintained an out-patient department. Some hospitals have had a very heavy emergency service, such as the l'Hôpital St Luc in Montreal, or the receiving hospitals in some American cities such as in Detroit. Others, and particularly smaller hospitals, had only an operating room, really a dressing room, with some ancillary facilities, staffed as needed and closed at night unless required.

Here, too, the picture has changed remarkably over these five decades. The internal combustion engine has seen to that. Cars are no longer put up on jacks in the garage for the winter to take the weight off the tires as was the common practice for 'pleasure cars' at the time of the first world war. The winter ploughing of roads, unheard of then, has been a normal procedure for some years; today the rural roads are more conducive to winter travel than are those of the cities. The horse on the farm has been replaced by the tractor and other motorized equipment and that means more accidents. Skiing has become a major winter sport with scores of clubs and with access to countless winterized cottages by means of ploughed highways and snowmobiles. There has been more night driving and drag racing. In addition to accidents, there have been more coronary attacks.

All of this means that practically every hospital no matter how small must be prepared for emergencies. The time-honored emergency door locked at night to keep out inebriates ('In case of emergency please ring the bell and wait') no longer meets the situation. For quite a few hospitals this has meant a twenty-four-hour service with an intern or resident, or perhaps, in the many hospitals without interns, a younger staff man provided with a room and bed in the department. Planners must now provide a much larger department with more dressing or operative areas, a twenty-four-hour staff, a bedroom for the staff man (or intern) on night duty and, desirably, an observation or holding area for patients with head injury and other potentially serious problems. The X-ray facilities are planned to be adjacent (or a portable machine is kept available) and, as discussed above, the non-admitted minor-procedure unit should also be adjacent and use some of the same ancillary facilities.

The Non-Emergency Ambulatory Patient
This is an ambulatory type of patient which has increased tremendously in recent years and has complicated the picture for the hospital organizer who likes to have everything classified and clear cut. This is the patient who has a headache 'or sumpin,' is not seriously ill but turns up at the hospital at any hour of the evening or night and wants service. In the 'old days' nobody in smaller towns ever thought of going to the hospital directly for the odd ache or pain. They either sought their own doctor or made the rounds of the offices by phone (if they had one) or on foot. In those days the doctors' offices were usually in the doctors' homes, often reasonably grouped together in the better residential area and yet not far from the business district and the off-the-street driving sheds where the farmers usually left their teams content with nose bags and a forkful of hay. In larger centres where many newcomers had no personal physician, patients frequently did go to emergency but not to the extent that they do now. If the hospital had an out-patient department and the supervisor did not think the patient was threatened with 'impending dissolution' (to borrow a phrase from the old textbooks on angina pectoris), she politely but firmly referred him to the clinic next day or later in the week.

This increased turning to the hospital for emergency and non-emergency consultation has not been without justification. This is particularly evident in the evenings, during the night and over weekends. Doctors no longer have their offices in their homes (the car in the drive used to be a dead give-away that the doctor was home); it is exceedingly difficult to get a doctor at all over weekends; doctors may not list their home phones and the answering services are most protective; and, if a doctor is finally located, he is very likely to refer the patient to the hospital anyway.

The logical conclusion is for the patient to head for the hospital without wasting time and that has become an increasingly common practice. Wednesday afternoon coverage is usually arranged by the practitioners in smaller centres but weekends and evenings are another matter. What applied to emergencies has applied more and more to the non-emergency out-patient. While most of such could wait without harm until their own doctor would be available or for the appropriate out-patient clinic, it seems to be in the air these days with 'instant' everything else to want instant service at the hospital in the middle of the night as well. Who can say that the pain in the abdomen or in the chest is not an emergency? We have all agreed that our emergency service, particularly at night and over weekends, is being abused, but how can the hospital personnel make the necessary decisions without such being made by a physician? Many experienced staff members feel that it is really not possible and that this is a development which may have to be accepted. The long-existing type of out-patient clinic has been declining in importance and patronage, except in a few instances. Because of these more recent developments, it will be merged probably into a general ambulatory-care area, covering non-admitted minor procedures and examinations, and drop-in or low-pay out-patients, with some segregation for traumatic emergencies.

This may be but additional evidence that the hospital is becoming the centre or hub of the health services of the area.

REGIONAL PLANNING

The hospital system in Canada, like so many other developments in this country, has been based on the concept of 'rugged individualism.' This applied whether the hospital was voluntary or municipal. The hospital board was charged with the responsiblity of providing whatever type of service or facility it deemed necessary and could provide within its budget.

This localization of responsiblity had much to commend it. The hospital was very much part of the community. When funds to provide new facilities or to renovate old ones were required, the money was raised locally, either by subscription or from local taxes, or both. The people felt a personal interest in their hospital and a responsiblity for it. The women's auxiliaries worked endlessly to achieve their objectives.

This localization also had its drawbacks. There was a focusing of attention on the more dramatic active treatment type of hospital, to the neglect of care for the chronically ill, or of the mentally ill, or of the aged and senile. In the active treatment hospital, there was a tendency to bypass the provision of facilities for psychiatric patients, for the alcoholic or the drug addict and even the responsibility for communicable disease patients. There was a tendency to take pride in having the best private floor or pavilion in the area; each hospital strove for the best operative suite, delivery suite or radiological equipment. What one hospital got, its neighbour felt compelled to duplicate; if it did not do so, it lost status in the eyes of the public, or, perhaps more correctly expressed, on the tip of its gossipy tongue. Many hospitals had equipment they could not adequately use, or use frequently enough to warrant the investment. One could name small rural hospitals with orthopaedic and other equipment more lavish than in some of the best teaching hospitals.

The result of this 'rugged individualism' was a remarkably adequate hospital system for most types of short illness or trauma, but with many gaps in the community's health coverage for its citizens. The boards tended to undertake what could be done within the four walls of the hospital and leave the remaining problems to others. We cannot blame them for this. They were giving freely of their time and substance for their institution without any earthly reward except the criticism of those who passed on third-hand tales of cold meals or delayed bed pans. They were doing more than their share of voluntary work and felt justified in leaving something to others. The basic weakness was the lack of an overall co-ordinated plan.

This did result, not only in regrettable gaps in our health program, but often in unnecessary and expensive duplication. This situation has been recognized for some time but we failed to evolve a method of dealing with it except in cancer therapy, where government assistance was the main factor in having this type of treatment concentrated in a few designated centres.

Quite a few provincial studies and surveys during the forties and fifties recommended planning and operation of hospital and health services on a regional basis. The opposition of local communities and hospital personnel, however, has on many occasions delayed progress. And even though hospital associations frequently divided into regional districts which met regularly – thereby keeping the members in each region informed of each other's services, both existing and planned – there was still a lack of incentive for them to co-ordinate those services.

Co-ordination came with the greater participation of the provincial governments in the financing of construction and operation. With the rising costs of construction as well as operation, governments have become vitally concerned with cost items, be they the quality of hinges or a new operative suite. With this crackdown on hospital construction expenditure, regional or area-wide planning became the order of the day. Unnecessary duplication of facilities in an area, or overemphasis upon one phase of care to the detriment of other essential levels or types of care, has now begun to be minimized. In several provinces, before the request of a hospital for approval of expansion or renovation is considered, a role study for the various hospitals in the region must be undertaken. This indicates what each hospital should be planning to provide in the future, what services can be duplicated in each active treatment hospital (for example, general medicine, general surgery) and which could be more efficiently concentrated in one or two only (for instance, cardiac surgery, brain surgery, renal dialysis, psychiatry, or, in some areas, obstetrics and/or children's diseases).

To facilitate regional planning a number of the provinces have set up regional planning councils to advise the provincial government as to which projects deserve approval. In some cases budget limitations force the regional councils to set project priorities. Nova Scotia, Ontario, Manitoba, Saskatchewan and British Columbia had set up such regional planning councils by 1970. Alberta was studying the advisability of such action and Quebec had included legislation providing for considerable decentralization of authority in the provision of all types of health services.

The extent to which regional planning councils should have executive and fund-raising powers has been debated a great deal. In making a study of area-wide requirements a few years ago for a large metropolitan centre, my associates and I found that the great majority of such regional councils across the continent, most being in the United States, did not have executive nor tax-fixing powers. The earlier metropolitan planning councils were set up to protect the big donors in the area from the stunning total of the many quite unrelated campaigns set up by individual hospitals. The potential donors found that this total over, say a ten-year period, could be drastically reduced and sometimes more than cut in half by paring off the unnecessary duplications. A favorable report by such a body could ensure the success of a campaign; an adverse report by such a body could quickly ruin it. No executive power was needed.

In Canada, the provincial governments provide most of the capital funds and this does affect the situtation. On the one hand, community and regional participation can take much of the political heat and pressure off the provincial authorities and remove the criticism that they do not understand the local situation. By giving substantial authority to such planning bodies the provincial government can ensure not only top calibre membership but also a much more effective role. Some regional council members with only advisory powers have pointed out, not infrequently, that hospital boards will go right to the government insurance authorities, the minister or the premier, and completely bypass the planning council in the process.

On the other hand, most provincial governments are reluctant to delegate authority and responsibility where such large sums of provincial revenues are involved. In any case the provinces believe that they would not be justified in giving executive power to regional councils, many of which are largely or completely made up of hospital board and staff representatives. It is difficult for them to maintain a proper perspective respecting the closing of a hospital or the creation of a new one. Even where the municipalities and the public have considerable representation on the planning councils, town rivalries in rural areas make it difficult for them to agree on a justifiable radical decision if it hurts or eliminates one of them.

Theoretically the majority of the council should be carefully chosen, public-spirited citizens not connected with any hospital and consequently relatively free of bias. They should be representative of the citizens of the region and rely on an advisory committee composed of medical and hospital personnel. The Greater Vancouver Hospital Region, established under the British Columbia Municipal Act, is set up along these lines. The British Columbia district councils have planning responsibilities along with the authority to recommend certain local taxes to help finance hospital construction; however, the total amount is limited and subject to referendum. The initial setting of priorities is the responsibility of the district councils, which handle the individual requests from hospitals. The councils are largely made up of local politicians and municipal officials and there has been a tendency to effect a wide distribution of funds so that each component area gets a slice. This has meant that it has sometimes been difficult to get widespread support for a much-needed major centralized development. In most cases, however, a considerable degree of objectivity has prevailed.

These councils do not have effective autonomy; their recommendations are subject to the scrutiny and approval of the provincial authorities. As in the rest of the country, so long as the provinces budget for and distribute such a large portion of capital costs, they will probably insist on having the final decision. Thus the future of regional planning councils depends not so much on the willingness of hospital, medical and community leaders to co-operate in planning for their regions (this is occasionally still a problem) but on the degree to which the provinces will be willing to decentralize their planning authority. If the recommendations of regional councils are continually ignored, deferred or drastically altered, they will simply wither and fade into the background, their members convinced they are wasting their time.

In recent years there have been recommendations to broaden the scope of hospital planning councils to include planning for all health activities that are financed primarily through tax revenues. These would include public-health services, homes for the aged, clinics, ambulance services, and home-care programs as well as hospital facilities.

8
Much still to be done

This chapter could not be begun more appropriately than with a comment made by one of the soundest leaders the hospital field has ever had.

Dr S.S. Goldwater of New York City was the first recognized hospital planning consultant in America. A number of Canadian hospitals profited immensely by his sage advice on planning or on operation from about 1910 until his death in 1942. He gained much public respect as director of the Mount Sinai Hospital in New York, by his extensive writings and, later, as the far-seeing commissioner of hospitals in that city. In 1908 he was president of the American Hospital Association when it first met in Toronto. Later, in the 1930s, he organized its various councils and their co-ordinating committee, this work being continued by Dr Michael Davis, who had founded the training program in hospital administration and whose text on the subject is still in use.

Towards the end of his tremendous career (and one suspects that he knew his months were limited) we were having lunch together in New York after his return from Moscow where he had been invited to review with the Russians a new type of hospital they proposed (which, by the way, Dr Goldwater discouraged as being too visionary and impracticable).

He asked me my age and remarked: 'You're twenty-two years younger than I am.' Then he laid his hand on my arm and said, very quietly: 'Harvey, I would give everything I have if I could just set the calendar back those twenty-odd years. There is so much to be done and so little time.' Dr Goldwater, like so many in the hospital field, never wasted time and his contributions are as valid today as when they were written.

HOSPITAL INFECTIONS

While hospital infections in general are not as dangerous today as they were before the contributions of Pasteur, Lister and Semmellweis, they are still a constant menace. They are probably a greater menace than we realize for many infections are obscure, of varying symptomatology, persistent and very resistant to treatment. The security we have felt in recent years, first with sulfa and similar drugs and then with the antibiotics, has been shaken sadly as we find the causative organisms becoming more resistant to drugs and antibiotics and as new viruses are identified which pay little attention to our defensive weapons.

Researchers in the field of hospital infections like Dr Carl Walters and Dr Feingold of Boston, Dr Bertha Litsky at the University of Massachusetts and Dr Reinarz at the University of Dallas have demonstrated repeatedly the infective danger of many of the systems used in present-day hospitals. Among the potential contaminators are ventilation, air circulation and humidification, various clinical procedures, and equipment involving re-use of equipment such as nebulizers and catheters. The researchers have pointed out the hazards inherent in poorly dried mops, floor cleaning methods, cracked terrazzo, medication and other carts, bedside carafes, faucet aerators, urinals, toilet bowls, solution bottles and more recently the indiscriminate and overly enthusiastic use of carpeting. Nosocomial infections may not be as obvious as in the days of erysipelas, typhoid, and home-sterilized solutions, but the subtle and less-easily detected infections of the present time may be equally virulent. Carriers of pseudomonas and other infections may be staff members, in which case they can be detected; if they are patients the task is more difficult. Much has been done to point out the danger areas and to control the situation, but much more remains to be done.

Many larger hospitals have committees of the medical staff to check unexplained or recurrent infections, usually suture breakdowns, but their responsibility goes much further than is usually recognized. The day may come soon when the hospital commissions will authorize the employment of a highly trained individual to direct controls for hospitals in an area and probably have all the laboratory work done by specially trained and interested bacteriologists.

RURAL COVERAGE

The problem of the rural hospital will need considerable study. Over the years we have had much better coverage than most countries with extensive rural areas. In the east generally and in British Columbia, the voluntary hospitals plus the Red Cross outpost hospitals have provided a reasonably satisfactory network. The Prairie provinces have developed rural municipal hospitals, Saskatchewan featuring 'union' hospitals supported by several municipalities. In Newfoundland the isolated outposts have been built by the provincial government and by the International Grenfell Association.

The picture, however, is changing. Medicine is developing so rapidly that it is becoming very difficult for the small hospital to provide up-to-date scientific diagnosis and treatment for its patients. Where the small hospital manages today it is often because of having laboratory and radiological services provided by a nearby large hospital. With paved roads, winter snow-ploughing and good care there has been a tendency sometimes for the concerned patient to go directly to a larger centre, thus making it harder for the local doctor and the small hospital to maintain good service. Saskatchewan developed too many rural hospitals in the forties and has been trying to close down a number of them, a slow process due to local opposition. It is a widely appreciated axiom that one hospital of one hundred beds is able to give better service in any given area than two of fifty beds, even if some of the patients must drive a few miles further. Likewise, for some areas, one hospital of two hundred beds can give more efficient service than two of one hundred each.

This, however, does not mean that small rural hospitals do not fulfil a necessary function, In a country like Canada, with isolated communities stretching from the mountain valleys of British Columbia to the isolated outposts of Newfoundland and Labrador, some hospital provision is essential. In fact many of these communities could not attract nor hold a doctor without such facilities. This was a basic reason behind the rash of small hospitals developed in the Prairie provinces before and after the second world war. For most illnesses or injuries the usual facilities of the small hospital are reasonably adequate. For quite a few emergencies the presence of a rural hospital, where hemorrhage can be arrested, shock overcome and other emergency treatment given, can save many lives. If the technique is good, it should be better for the maternity patient and the baby in the hospital than in the farmhouse.

The answer may well be the development of a system of care which would include rural hospitals but a smaller number of them. More outpost nursing stations in sparsely settled areas could be manned by nurses, prepared to give emergency care (one to three beds) preliminary to sending on to a hospital, but not so set up as to encourage the patient to stay by thinking he was now in hospital. Alberta had a system of this nature some years ago. The Red Cross nursing outposts have demonstrated the value of this arrangement, as have also the stations established by the Grenfell Mission in Labrador.

The flying doctor system developed by the Reverend John Flynn in New South Wales, Australia, proved to be an excellent solution for sparsely settled areas. The ranchers, at least in the early thirties, sent out a call in Morse code with a foot-operated generator and the flying doctor came, gave treatment and, if necessary, took the patient back with him to the base. Saskatchewan was the first province in this country to have a government-operated flying ambulance service. Air transportation is now used in many parts of Canada, but mostly on an emergency basis. (Helicopters are even used in and near cities to avoid the weekend traffic tie-up.)

For those rural hospitals set up in more thickly populated rural areas – Nova Scotia, Prince Edward Island and southern Ontario, for example – other steps should be considered. From my own experience, the greatest factor holding them back from attaining their full potential is their almost complete lack of functional relationships. Only now are some of these larger rural hospitals becoming involved in regional planning councils. They work alone; their staffs often retain patients who should be hospitalized in a better equipped and staffed urban hospital; and they often endeavor to overcome this lack of facilities by installing pieces of equipment which they are not staffed to use properly or which they cannot use often enough to warrant the expenditure involved. They are sometimes suspicious of rural area-wide planning because they fear that they will get the 'chronics' and the other fellow the 'interesting' services. Even old hockey rivalries may becloud the situation. Manitoba tried some years back, when the Honorable Ivan Schulz was minister of health, to assign facilities of varying size (down to eight beds) to various towns and villages in a well-thought-out plan to provide coverage yet avoid unnecessary duplication, but the plan was scuttled by the political pressure put upon the cabinet by the 'have-not' communities which could not see a neighboring but better-located town get thirty-five beds (and an X-ray) compared to their, say, fifteen beds.

There is a definite need for more thinking in proper perspective. A rural hospital may really be needed and certain services should be provided: emergency obstetrics, general medicine, minor and the less complicated or exacting major surgery. With a well-qualified (certified) surgeon on the staff the extent of coverage can be much widened, and so with other specialists. But some rural hospitals are only a few minutes apart in motoring time. It would be much better for the community to have one better-equipped obstetrical and neo-natal service in the area and one children's service. One emergency only should be kept open all night. Only one need have a special room for alcoholics or for emotionally disturbed patients to be transferred elsewhere later.

For years many smaller hospitals have shared the services of part-time radiologists and pathologists. This has brought expert diagnostic service to these hospitals. Some have made arrangements with larger hospitals in the area for accounting services and sometimes for group purchasing. The sharing of services could be increased considerably if the principle could be extended by means of a comprehensive tie-in of a small and a large hospital – a form of 'big brother' relationship. This could mean more readily obtained advice on a host of medical matters, on nursing procedures, on administrative principles and details, and on the problems of individual departments – dietary, housekeeping, pharmacy and so forth. Special equipment could be loaned and diagnostic tests more readily arranged. If desired, there could be interlocking boards. All of this would mean greater service to the rural patient and he could still, in most instances, remain under his family physician.

The most difficult hurdle to overcome in fully bringing this broader service to the non-urban patient is the basis of medical remuneration. As long as doctors must provide for their families they are going to be reluctant, under the present fee system, to turn over their patients to someone else unless the case is obviously one needing someone else's skill. Great Britain tried to solve this problem with the 'panel' system, each practitioner receiving an annual amount for the patients on his panel. While it has proven effective, as shown by national health statistics, it has been criticized severely by many in the profession. One wonders if there would have been as much – or any appreciable – criticism if the annual financial return had been as lucrative as is possible under the medical insurance plans in this country. Without question this factor will need to be resolved satisfactorily before the problem of rural hospital care can be settled.

The solution, too, must ensure a sufficient income to the rural practitioner so that good doctors will be willing to undertake such practice and also be happy professionally, preferably by bringing them into the orbit of the urban medical staff members to compensate for the more frequent turning over of their more serious cases.

THE TEAM CONCEPT

In view of the improbability of solving the increasing shortage of rural practitioners under our present system and the staggering costs of added medical schools, it is apparent that some radical changes will need to be made in our methods of delivering health care to these vital areas. A 'team' concept is essential. This cannot be achieved, except in a superficial manner, unless the key members of the team – the doctors – are willing to unbend from their traditional participation as individual contractors and enter fully into the comprehensive program for the provision of all health services in the area.

There is nothing new about this concept; it has been demonstrated in 'emerging' countries, in mission centres and in Newfoundland, not only by the Grenfell organization but by the long-existing type of provincially sponsored medical care in many of the outposts. It does mean a willingness on the part of the profession to help develop, rather than keep aloof from, local and regional plans of this nature. It also means an effort by medical schools to stress the importance of helping to meet the community needs as well as to teach scientific knowledge and procedures.

We might learn a good deal from what is being done, for instance, in the medical school of Ahmadu Bello University of Zaria, Nigeria. Dr H. Scarborough, dean of medicine, noting the impossibility of even meeting the minimum ratio recommended by World Health Organization of one doctor per 5,000 population, has come to the conclusion that the solution lies in a 'health team' as the fundamental unit, rather than individual doctor. The doctor would head the team and would have as associates two general 'clinical auxiliaries,' one or two maternal and child welfare auxiliaries, one minor surgical/anaesthetic auxiliary, and one laboratory diagnosis auxiliary.

Such a team would be based at a rural health centre. The team would supplement the work of dispensary attendants and provide some of the medical care in branch dispensaries associated with the health centre. The centre, in turn, would be related to a community hospital. The medical school tries to provide some of its training in an environment not too different from what the graduate may face later. (This is somewhat comparable to the use here of family practice units in teaching hospitals to acquaint the students with general practice.) The medical school also stresses 'the importance of, and the satisfaction to be obtained from, a medical practice outside the hospital environment and especially the value of training the doctor as part of the health team.'[1] The medical school is also responsible for the training of the 'medical auxiliaries.'

1 H. Scarborough, writing in *Newsletter No. 10* of the Teaching Hospital Group of the International Hospital Federation, April 1971. (Lloyd F. Detweiler of the University Health Service Hospital, University of British Columbia, has been chairman of this Teaching Hospital Group for several years.)

HOSPITAL PRIVILEGES

The future of hospital appointments will be subject to considerable re-examination in the next few years. The traditional basis, outlined previously in Chapter 4, has been accepted generally, particularly since the clarification of specialist qualification was achieved by the Royal College of Physicians and Surgeons of Canada. It was recognized that those members of the active staff who did the free work on the public wards and spent endless time on hospital committees with no remuneration had a reasonable prior claim on the private beds. Sometimes this was carried too far. Conditions are changing, however, and the old quite extensive 'free' work is now largely covered by medical insurance, welfare provision, workmen's compensation, automobile insurance or other coverage. In those hospitals with regulations whereby these accounts on the standard wards cannot be collected directly, they usually go into a special fund for later distribution to the staff as a whole or to certain specific projects. True, none of it may get back to the top men on the staff, but, again, an increasing number of them in teaching hospitals are on geographic full-time appointment with remuneration to cover many of their duties.

In keeping with the trend to challenge the status quo everywhere, those who want full privileges in their fields are becoming more and more vociferous. This poses quite a problem for hospital trustees. Traditionally the law requires the board of a hospital to exercise sound judgment in the appointment of doctors to the medical staff. The hospital may not be liable for the individual act of a doctor but it must have shown care and judgment in his appointment. Board members realize the problem of a doctor who needs a hospital connection to make effective application of his knowledge; they realize also that, with patients flocking to hospitals for non-emergency as well as emergency care, the hospital is really becoming the physician to the community. Nevertheless, because of the legal responsibility placed on them by law, trustees must retain some control over who gets hospital privileges and to what extent. Arbitrarily to take that responsibility from them would make their position untenable and might well result in numerous resignations.

Now they exercise this control by letting the credentials committee of the medical staff recommend approval or denial of appointments. The medical staff should be better judges of an application than a non-medical board and this is a sound procedure. The answer may be in a more liberal extension of staff privileges in some hospitals, always, of course, within the qualifications of the applicant. However, the automatic opening up of staff privileges to anyone with a license to practice, as desired by some, would create a chaotic situation which would not be in the interests of the patients. As for specialist work, certification is a safeguard but there is no piece of paper that can guarantee good judgment, control in a crisis, or ability to work with others.

IN LIEU OF INTERNS

The provision of medical assistance and of patient oversight, traditionally the areas covered by the interns and residents in the hospitals so favored, has been undergoing considerable change. At best only the active-treatment teaching hospitals and the better-known non-teaching hospitals have been reasonably sure of obtaining interns; the great majority of hospitals either do not have them at all; or may hire a few by advertising and paying well; or may be able to obtain intermittent service by reason of the local interests of the intern. Unless a hospital is approved for internship the likelihood of maintaining a service is very slim; even then there are more internships approved than there are potential interns. Since the second world war many refugee and immigrant doctors have been available for intern service but their number is now decreasing and, of course, they can only get credit for their license by serving in a hospital approved for internship.

In recent years the teaching hospitals have been accepting more and more interns and have been paying remuneration, a contrast from the days when a teaching hospital provided nothing but maintenance and uniforms. That made it harder for the non-teaching hospital. Now the trend is to do away with internships in the teaching hospitals in favour of final-year clinical clerks. The licensing bodies are taking a closer look at where the internship has been served. For instance, the College of Physicians and Surgeons of Quebec now requires that the internship be taken only in a hospital affiliated with a medical faculty. Some medical schools in the past provided the final year as an internship in a hospital approved by the school. The clinical clerkship is really an adaptation of that approach. Now the residencies, too, are being determined by the medical schools, rather than solely by the Royal College.

The decisions, naturally, are being made from the viewpoint of medical education, as they should be, but what of the desirability of providing a valuable service to the patients in the other larger hospitals, not to mention the smaller hospitals which exist in greater numbers?

This is a major problem that the hospitals and their staffs have not squarely faced. Medical procedures have developed so extensively that the doctor in charge cannot be expected to perform or attend to all of the technical procedures at the bedside. Nurses and operating-room technicians can be satisfactory assistants in the operating or delivery room and nurses are doing the monitoring and many of the nursing-floor procedures which a few years ago were considered quite beyond the scope of the nurse. Many are giving intramuscular and intravenous injections and other even more demanding treatment procedures. But there are still many procedures which the doctor is expected to do and these include the long essential compilation of the patients' clinical records, which the busy practitioner cannot ignore with the accreditation committee breathing down his neck.

Twenty or more years ago one of the large eastern states passed a law requiring hospitals above a minimum size to employ an intern for every one hundred beds. The concept was good but the law was completely impracticable. Even interpreting the requirement as a paid 'house physician' of retirement – or any – age, the law could not be enforced.

Obviously we must develop in hospitals another level of clinical personnel to meet the needs of the other 90 percent and over of the hospitals. This must be a person who can perform the many minor clinical procedures of a technical nature in the hospital; who can write family and personal history and all but the physical examination of the patient's history; who can cut down on a vein if necessary, control progressive treatments, or remove stitches; who can, if necessary in smaller hospitals, do emergency simple laboratory procedures. Some of this is being done now by skilled nurses and by technicians, but the undertakings should be extended. The individuals concerned could have background either as nurse or as technician. They could be known as 'clinical assistants' or some other appropriate name. Schools could be developed for their specialized training, just as we now train inhalation therapists or operating-room technicians. The trend today is to take training for many activities in colleges, but this seems to be a type of training best given in an active-treatment hospital. Had this been a problem of the large teaching hospitals, it would have been solved long ago, but it must be solved soon in the interests of the other hospitals where a ready solution is not so apparent.

PHYSICIANS' ASSISTANTS

Such a nursing-floor assistant should not be confused with the 'physicians' assistants' or 'medical assistants' strongly urged by some at the present time to relieve the practising doctor of many of his less exacting duties in conducting his practice.

The physicians' or medical assistants could have hospital duties somewhat comparable to the requirements for 'clinical assistants.' However, in the main, discussions with regard to this type of person have centred about an individual who would be employed by one physician, or one group, and have duties more closely related to office practice or home visits than hospital activities.

Doctors have had the benefit of competent office assistance for many years. Office assistants with a nurses' training could be of more clinical help than those without, although, irrespective of background, many have become quite competent in various clinical duties. But now the public is becoming interested. If doctors cannot make house calls because of lack of time, or it takes up to five or six weeks to get an office appointment, efficiency-minded people are asking if too much of the doctor's time is being wasted on work that could be done quite adequately by someone with less public money invested in his training. The Russians have been filling the gap with partially trained *feldschers*. In the United States, the classification is recognized by the federal civil service commission; there are six college courses approved and six pending; some one hundred training programs have been listed; there is an American Association of Medical Assistants with its own certifying board; the AMA has given it substantial monetary assistance. The Board on Medicine of the National Academy of Sciences recognizes three types of physicians' assistants, types A, B, and C, evaluated according to their qualifications. Type A can operate on occasion without the immediate surveillance of the physician and can exercise a degree of independent judgment.

This development in the United States is summarized here because there has been considerable discussion on the subject in Canada. While most of the discussion here has related to the employment of physicians' assistants in office and home duties, their special training, if comparable to that being developed in the United States, might well qualify them for clinical work in hospitals, along the lines discussed in the preceding section. There they are trained to handle a wide range of equipment – ECG, defibrillators, and so forth – and even to do physical examinations, which is going a long way. Some advocates here would set up a distinct category of 'practitioner associate' with a four-year course of training, less credit for nursing or other related training. It is thought that the majority qualifying would have a nursing background.

However, the nursing profession is opposed to the idea of setting up still another category. In 1970, the CNA board of directors, in a statement to the then federal Minister of Health, John Munro, asserted that health needs could be served effectively and economically by expanding the role of the nurse. It would be less costly to provide short courses for nurses than to fund programs to train a totally new category.

Present courses in Canada are quite limited. The School of Nursing at Dalhousie, Nova Scotia, has an outpost-nursing program, a two-year course for graduate nurses. It leads to accreditation for complete midwifery, public-health nursing and basic medical and surgical clinic practice. The objective is to prepare for independent roles in the remote regions of Canada's north country. This course has been financed by the medical services branch of the federal Department of National Health and Welfare. The other course is the advanced obstetrical nursing program at the University of Alberta.

Many problems will need to be clarified in the development of these 'general practice associates' irrespective of whether they work in hospitals. All provincial medical acts will need revising. Not the least difficulty will be that of medico-legal responsibility. Leaving a situation with a less trained individual might be construed as negligence. If the general practice associates are legally permitted to act independently in some situations, where is the line to be drawn? However, these matters seldom create trouble in a doctor-nurse relationship, or with a technologist or a radiographer. The use of medical assistants and clinical assistants as outlined above will have to advance slowly and carefully, however, as far as hospitals are concerned, for lawsuits and public outcry in press, radio and TV would be loud if something went seriously wrong with a hospitalized patient due to error of these medical or clinical assistants and the hospital would be held accountable.

THE HOSPITAL AS CENTRE OF THE AREA'S HEALTH PROGRAM

Previously, reference was made to the increased use of hospitals for ambulatory care as further evidence of the hospital becoming the centre of the health care program of the area. There is ever-mounting evidence that this is becoming a fact. For several decades medical practice has become more and more centred in hospitals; teaching hospitals have many geographic full-time appointees on their staffs; medical office buildings are being located as close to hospitals as possible. The clinical role of hospitals is becoming much broader as new services or undertakings are added. More educational programs and more research are taking place in hospitals. More local offices of specialty organizations are being located in hospitals or immediately adjacent – agencies relating to cancer, arthritis, crippled children, home nursing (VON), and public health offices among others.

In the late thirties and forties, the W.K. Kellogg Foundation urged using the active treatment hospital as a health program centre in Canada and the United States. This foundation accomplished a great deal across the country under the stimulus created by Graham Davis. He, himself, would like to have achieved more, but these movements do take time to grow. Some medium-sized communities with public health nurses located them in the hospital with good results. In centres large enough to have a full-time medical health officer, however, he and his inspectors liked to be downtown – where they could be readily available for consultation with municipal officers, to carry out health examinations on food handlers, to handle milk inspection and the many other duties of the health department – and all too often the hospital was located away from the municipal offices and the downtown area.

With the general public becoming increasingly aware of medical technology and procedures, and with the emphasis on medical subjects on radio and TV, in magazine articles and in newspaper reports, more progress should be made in the seventies. Certainly the public is demanding more and better health facilities and government health insurance makes medical services more readily available to every family and individual.

Rather than simply reacting to the changes in medicine and society which are obliging the hospital to take on the role of health centre, the hospital should assume a greater responsibility for not only adjusting to, but also directing and encouraging a much broader function for itself. Regional planning bodies could be enlarged to work out more co-operation, not only between the hospitals of an area, but among all the bodies or agencies relating to health (and welfare too) in the area.

EXTRA-MURAL SERVICES

We are moving quickly into an era when the hospital, to fulfil its destiny, must reach out beyond its walls to better serve its community. Dignified isolation on a hilltop site no longer meets the needs of a changing era. As has been said aptly, emphasis is shifting to the care of the vertical patient.

This is not a sudden realization, for phases of the movement have been evident in various ways. A number of hospitals have participated actively in home-care programs. A few have had secondary divisions, for instance the former western division of the Montreal General Hospital and the Nora F. Henderson division of the Hamilton General Hospital. Some have participated in public health clinics other than in the hospital. Some have maintained close relations with outpost nursing units in outlying areas. But with the tremendous surge in urbanization and the problems of transportation for conventional out-patients, new urban situations are arising. An increasing number of people in this transient age do not have a family physician and sometimes cannot get one even if they try. More and more, either on its own volition or with the approval of a physician, the public is seeking the facilities of the hospital not so much as indigents or with token payments (although that still continues to an increasing extent), but as paying, insured patients.

There is a growing realization that hospitals can best meet this need by going into the community themselves with clinics and dispensaries. 'Storefront' clinics are beginning to appear in slum areas, shopping centres and even office buildings. Better and fuller contacts can be made by bringing such facilities as can be moved closer to the people. A number of hospitals in the United States have made these steps. For instance, one has converted an old convent into a community clinic. One has a converted trailer equipped for various services. Another has set up a million dollar suburban clinic. Several of these facilities operate on a prepayment membership basis, a feature no longer applicable in Canada. Clinics have been opened in high-rise apartments for elderly citizens as part of a welfare and recreational program. Hospital facilities are being used for 'meals on wheels' services to shut-ins. Community comprehensive programs are involving hospital services and skills as well as welfare and recreation services.

These skills and facilities are needed in the inner city as well as in new suburban areas and, equally so, in sparsely settled areas. A recent example of the downtown type of service is the clinic St Michael's Hospital has opened in the Commerce Court office complex in Toronto. It is being run by St Michael's staff who provide diagnostic and emergency services. A physiotherapy clinic and pharmacy are also included. The Toronto Western Hospital is planning to open a clinic in the new Metro Centre that is to be built on Toronto's waterfront.

Related to these extra-mural services is the emphasis on health maintenance organizations (Health Maintenance Organization), a movement first sponsored by the American Hospital Association in 1969 to 1970 and then taken up by the Nixon administration. The emphasis, as the name suggests, is on health maintenance rather than acute episodic care. By contracting with the federal government to provide all health maintenance services to its enrollees through a fixed-fee arrangement, and with the co-operation of medical and hospital personnel, suppliers and consumers of health care share the risks of ill health. Incentives are provided for all concerned to control costs through a greater emphasis on preventive medicine, community clinics, rehabilitative care and other measures to ensure that the number of patients receiving active treatment hospital care is controlled. Experience has shown that the quality of care sponsored by HMO's has not deteriorated. There have been fewer premature births and infant deaths and a longer lifespan for elderly patients as compared to other more conventional health delivery systems. Hospital councils, medical societies and schools, Blue Cross plans, and private physician group practices have all shown great interest in operating comprehensive health maintenance organizations. A training program, mostly for Blue Cross and other hospital insurance personnel, has been set up by Kaiser-Permanente in California and the Health Insurance Plan of New York.

TLC

Because of the many and increasing factors which tend to make hospital care more and more impersonal, many members of the hospital fraternity often wonder to what extent we shall be able to retain the traditional spirit of hospitals – that atmosphere of tender loving care (TLC). Sister M. Berthe Dorais, SGM, of St Boniface, in a recent letter to me wrote:

The hospital people of the past half century were concerned above all else with *patient* care, relying on personal communications more than on technological skills still in their infancy, as compared with today's complex medical center. Will such a basic human approach filled with awe for the dignity of the human person survive the new age of computerized medicine?

The age of computerized medicine involves more than computers and, in the sense used here, it began a decade or more ago. Increased use of the hospitals for less serious conditions, encouraged by the complexity of medicine and the lowering of the financial barrier by Blue Cross and then hospital insurance; early ambulation and shorter average stay; increasing automation; movement of patients from intensive care, to normal service, often to convalescent or chronic care units; confusion of the patient by a daily parade of several laboratory technicians, each for a different purpose; maids who cannot speak English (or French); the endless parade of strange plumbers, electricians, electronics men for TV, radio or two-way call systems, window adjusters, curtain changers, strange nurses and stranger interns – a parade of often over twenty-five to thirty by actual count; a strange harassed voice over the two-way voice call system instead of a warm smile and the touch of an understanding hand; corridor voice call systems too loud or badly located; an increasing number of clockwatchers in spirit with the times; an increasing attitude on the part of some personnel that this is only a job, not an opportunity for dedicated service.

The patient often gets the impression that he is just a number. Our very efforts to preserve his individuality may be misconstrued – the elaborate and careful recording of all pertinent information in triplicate or more, and use of identification bands for adults as well as for the newborn. Hospital costs have risen tremendously, as noted earlier, and present-day administrators, like their predecessors, are striving to effect savings to keep the costs from skyrocketing. Time for the good old get-acquainted chats between patients and personnel is gone. If we are going to effect cures never before thought possible, veritably work miracles as the present-day hospital does daily, and do so at a cost that the economy can bear, some less essential services or refinements will have to go. The dweller in the modern urban apartment recalls with nostalgia the big lilac trees flanking the old home in the village and the hollyhocks along the board fence, but he knows he had to give up that life to have his present conveniences and way of life.

There are in our midst some whose imagination soars far into the misty future. And who knows, they may be right, as witness Jules Verne. They foresee the incoming patient, after being questioned and then anaesthetized or perhaps hypnotized, placed upon a conveyor system. As he progresses he gets urine and other checks, X-rays, provides biopsy specimens, then is completely exsanguinated and his blood replaced temporarily by a special fluid. His blood gets all necessary tests and is freed of harmful substances. Worn-out organs are replaced. His brain is re-tuned to improved performance (including memory), and psychiatric and emotional disturbances are corrected by electronic, sonar or laser treatment. Finally, he is re-assembled with his own purified or replacement blood, given final inspection, awakened, clothed and sent home – presumably with a twelve-month guarantee.

Until such developments occur, when patients would be treated like computer punch cards, to what extent can we preserve much of the spirit and atmosphere of the hospital of yesterday?

We can do a great deal. The board can start by selecting an administrator who is interested in human relations as well as in the colors of ink. The administrator can let it be known, and repeatedly, that every staff member, whether or not he ever sees a patient, must keep constantly in mind that the primary purpose of the hospital is to serve its patients, and that those who have to do with patients are expected to treat them with kindness, cheerfulness and consideration. Relatives and the public should be treated with courtesy. If they demonstrate that such courtesy is not warranted, they should be referred to the administrative staff. The switchboard operators should be given special tests for aptitude under tension. So should some interns and some supervisors. Medical students and often their demonstrators need to learn a lot about 'bedside manner.' Student nurses should learn early that they are also training to become actresses; no matter how tired or depressed or irate they may feel, they must always present a smile, a buoyant and sympathetic voice and a spirit of understanding and encouragement to the apprehensive and dejected patient.

Every effort must be made to maintain the interest of voluntary workers. They supply something to the spirit of a hospital that no others can provide. The hospital auxiliary with its many services can be of inestimable assistance and its work should be given every encouragement. Candystripers and other junior volunteers bring added sunshine to the wards. Service clubs, musical organizations, entertainers – all like to do something for hospital patients. They add a dimension to therapy that cannot be overestimated, for they are a continuing demonstration that somebody cares and that the patient is not just a number.

WHAT OF THE FUTURE?

In the future there will still be hospitals – that is, if an atomic war has not blasted human life off of this earth. While many diseases will have been conquered, including most forms of cancer, there will still be accidents, probably in increased number, and an increased proportion of the tissue breakdown or catabolic diseases. These will be of the heart, the arterial system, the kidneys, the liver and other organs. Obstetrics will continue at a reduced level but, as now, almost entirely in hospital or 'in transit.'

Hospitals will no longer operate as unrelated entities. Their development will be on a co-ordinated basis, overall community need determining their location, size and type of service undertaken. Regional boards or committees will make these recommendations to provincial controlling bodies. Major financing will be at the levels of the senior governments, but there should still be a place for voluntary finance and service within specific areas and directions.

The present gaps in our hospital and institutional care, largely in the less dramatic or appealing areas, will have been overcome with more adequate government financing and sponsorship. There will be a closer relationship between the various types and levels of care in hospitals and homes, resulting in more ready transfer and more efficiency. Rural hospitals will be linked with urban hospitals for the ready transfer of patients, for skilled medical assistance and for help in the problems of daily maintenance.

The number of beds required will not have increased at the rate experienced in recent years. Admissions will be much more rigidly controlled than at present. Patients requiring diagnostic study by hospital personnel using the extensive equipment and facilities which will continue to be centred in hospitals will not be admitted unless seriously ill or bed-confined. The majority of the patients will be looked after on an ambulatory non-admitted basis, reporting to the hospital at prescribed times for various tests and examinations. For patients who are from out-of-town or for whom transportation is difficult, most hospitals of any size will have nearby low-cost hostel accommodation.

This means that the diagnostic services will have become still more extensive than they are now, particularly the laboratories and radiology. The hospitals, particularly selected ones in strategic locations, will have become 'diagnostic centres.' The outpatient departments will have ceased to be operated for low-income patients in the neighbourhood and will have become the focal point for the disposition of large numbers of insurance-covered patients.

In addition to the non-admitted care of patients requiring diagnosis, hospitals will continue, as now, the care of non-admitted patients requiring various forms of treatment best provided by hospitals, but the extent of such care will increase. This will apply to physical therapy, occupational therapy and other forms of rehabilitation, shock treatments and various specialized procedures.

As for medical skills and knowledge, it is generally agreed that more advances have been made in the past hundred years than in all the centuries since the dawn of civilization. The tempo of this increase has been markedly accentuated during the past twenty-five years; therefore, it is logical to believe that the advances of the next century will far exceed what we can possibly forecast today. Our limited present-day replacement of skin, bone, blood vessels, kidneys, teeth, corneal tissue, et cetera, and the implantation of artificial joints, aortas and heart valves are proud achievements of the medical profession, but they will probably seem quite elementary a hundred years hence. The use of implanted battery-operated apparatus of miniature proportions to regulate the heart beat and the use of the 'artificial kidney' will certainly lead to other achievements.

Patients will be admitted for much more extensive overhaul and, if necessary, organ replacement. We can foresee patients being exsanguinated and their blood replaced, not by steady fresh blood replenishment, as we have been doing on infants for years, but by an almost complete blood withdrawal and temporary replacement by a highly complex fluid. The blood could be thoroughly checked, filtered free of chemical impurities and undesirable cells, enriched with desirable radioactive or other additives, and then replaced. A much more extensive replacement of worn-out or sclerosed tissue by other tissue, either of a synthetic nature or salvaged from other patients at death, will be possible. Possibly the factors limiting the use of tissue from lower animals and from most humans, which cause the transplanted tissue to be digested as a foreign body, will have been overcome, thus widening greatly the scope of replacement surgery.

Non-explosive anaesthetics will have come into general use. A greater use of cryography, or the marked lowering of body temperature, will permit more extensive and less hurried operations on the body, taking advantage of the much reduced level of the body metabolism, a state somewhat akin to that of animal hibernation. Induction of the hypnotic state may become much more widely practised, in some cases as a form of anaesthesia, in others as a form of treatment in neuroses and in various psychotic states.

Procedures now only suggested by animal research may become part of the regular work of the future hospital. For instance, the research claims that certain nucleic acids found in all living species, ribonucleic acid (RNA) and deoxyribonucleic acid (DNA), are the seat of memory and that memory can be transplanted by the transfer of certain brain or other tissue open interesting possibilities for biochemical studies and surgical procedures. Hormone transplants and extract injections will probably have their day and be replaced by synthetic substances. If nuclear explosions are not outlawed, or if contamination by contact with nuclear products in civilian life becomes common, selected hospitals will likely be designated to treat contaminated individuals.

Automation will increase tremendously. This will apply to diagnostic procedures, various forms of treatment, the many forms of communication within the hospital, records and statistics, power, air conditioning and treatment, et cetera. Undoubtedly there will still be exasperating and, at times, disastrous breakdowns and failures as now. Because these will probably involve the more complicated facets of automation, correction without delay will pose increasing problems, particularly for hospitals remote from the larger centres. It may be a factor in the concentration of hospital facilities, except those for emergency and relatively simple care, in centres rather than in rural areas. This could well result in the greater use of airlift to bring in patients from remote or isolated areas.

Automation will have a distinct effect on personnel. Many categories of staff will require much more technical knowledge of the equipment they are using. This will apply particularly to the technical staff, the nurses and the engineering staff. Special training will be required for many groups or individuals. A current problem, which will be greatly increased in the future, is that of actual danger to patients and operators through mishap in handling equipment involving various types of electrical currents. This will undoubtedly lead to requirements for more adequate training of all persons using this equipment, probably controlled by more adequate legislation and by licensure of individuals. Although it may be thought that automation should reduce personnel (and it will in one sense), this will be offset by the constant increase in the volume and scope of work with patients and on their hospital climatic environment.

Food service may be drastically changed. Almost all hospitals now do their own buying and cooking with a very few using outside caterers. Many believe that hospital food in the future will be largely prepared by outside firms, be pre-cooked and frozen, be received as individual portions, and be given final heating in the hospital in 'radar' heaters. This is now being done in some hospitals in California and in many restaurants elsewhere. Ever-changing special diets do complicate the picture in hospitals, but it is not difficult to foresee economies and not too much loss in flexibility through use by hospitals of such outside food services. This may be long in coming in smaller centres, but is feasible in large centres.

Finally, what of planning and construction? At the present time hospitals are almost always 'custom' planned to meet the special needs of the community, or the site, or the special requirements of the staff. This does add to the cost, but is justified because seldom do two hospitals require exactly the same facilities, particularly as most planning projects are extensions to existing hospitals rather than completely new ones.

Is it possible to look forward to the day when a computer, given the population of the area and the existing facilities, could come up immediately with the number of beds, the extent of operating rooms, the area of the emergency department, et cetera? Many believe so and are confident that the computer can even provide the plans. However, it is not quite that simple and indicates immaturity of thought.

Some advances are quite possible and can be anticipated long before the next hundred years pass. For instance, the adoption of a planning module, say, four feet, could result in all rooms or space being multiples of four feet in width. This could lead to considerable pre-fabrication of structures and to the planning of laboratory and other equipment to fit such rooms. There would be some drawbacks. For instance, suppose a room should be ideally thirteen or fourteen feet wide; twelve feet would be too little and sixteen would be wasteful of space. Undoubtedly, however, sufficient economies could result to warrant such a basis of planning. Cheaper materials will be developed and simplified methods of construction will be found. Considerable standardization will develop in the interests of economy.

To anticipate complete standardization on the basis of size would be anything but progress. To know the 'average' requirement is always of interest and usually helpful, but, in the case of a hospital, details must vary with the nature of the community, its growth, the particular qualifications and the 'drawing power' of the medical staff, the proximity and facilities of neighboring hospitals and other factors. Moreover, it has been our experience that specifications for hospitals become amazingly obsolete within a few years, even months, and accumulated data must be constantly screened and often discarded. A rigid form of standardization could follow the present and increasing reliance upon formulae in estimating need and in planning, but should it so happen, the necessity of swinging back to make the project fit the need will also become evident.

Appendixes

The Minimum Standard

for approval under the Hospital Standardization Program of the American College of Surgeons

1
That physicians and surgeons privileged to practice in the hospital be organized as a definite group or staff. Such organization has nothing to do with the question as to whether the hospital is 'open' or 'closed', nor need it affect the various types of staff organization. The word 'staff' is here defined as the group of doctors who practise in the hospital inclusive of all groups such as the 'regular staff' and the 'associate staff'.

2
That membership upon the staff be restricted to physicians and surgeons who are (a) full graduates of medicine of an acceptable medical school with the degree of Doctor of Medicine, in good standing and legally licensed to practise in their respective states or provinces; (b) competent in their respective fields and (c) worthy in character and in matters of professional ethics; that in this latter connection the practice of the division of fees, under any guise whatsoever, be prohibited.

3
That the staff initiate and, with the approval of the governing board of the hospital, adopt rules, regulations and policies governing the professional work of the hospital; that these rules, regulations and policies specifically provide:

a) That staff meetings be held at least once a month. (In large hospitals the departments may choose to meet separately.)

b) That the staff review and analyse at regular intervals their clinical experience in the various departments of the hospital, such as medicine, surgery, obstetrics and the other specialties; the clinical records of patients, free and pay, to be the basis of such review and analysis.

4
That accurate and complete records be written for all patients and filed in an accessible manner in the hospital – a complete case record being one which includes identification data; complaint; personal and family history; history of present illness; physical examination; special examinations, such as consultations, clinical laboratory, X-ray and other examinations; provisional or working diagnosis; medical or surgical treatment; gross and microscopial pathological findings; progress notes; final diagnosis; condition on discharge; follow-up and, in case of death, autopsy findings.

5
That diagnostic and therapeutic facilities under competent supervison be available for the study, diagnosis and treatment of patients, these to include at least (a) a clinical laboratory providing chemical, bacteriological, serological and pathological services; (b) an X-ray Department providing radiographic and fluoroscopic services.

Federal Health Officers

A. HEALTH MINISTERS

Department of Health, founded in 1919

Hon Newton W. Rowell	Aug 2, 1919–July 10, 1920
Hon James A. Calder	July 10, 1920–Sept 20, 1921
Hon John W. Edwards	Sept 21, 1921–Dec 29, 1921
Hon Henri S. Beland	Dec 29, 1921–April 14, 1926
Hon John C. Elliott	April 15, 1926–June 28, 1926
Hon R.J. Manion	June 29, 1926–July 12, 1926
Hon Eugene E. Paquet	Aug 23, 1926–Sept 25, 1926
Hon James H. King	Sept 25, 1926–June 18, 1930

Department of Pensions and National Health, formed in 1928

Hon Murray MacLaren	Aug 7, 1930–Nov 16, 1934
Hon Donald M. Sutherland	Nov 17, 1934–Oct 23, 1935
Hon Charles G. Power	Oct 23, 1935–Sept 18, 1939
Hon Ian A. MacKenzie	Sept 19, 1939–Oct 12, 1944

Department of National Health and Welfare, formed in 1944

Hon Brooke Claxton	Oct 13, 1944–Dec 11, 1946
Hon Paul Martin	Dec 12, 1946–June 21, 1957
Hon J. Waldo Monteith	Aug 22, 1957–April 22, 1963
Hon Julia V. Lamarsh	April 22, 1963–Dec 18, 1965
Hon Allan J. MacEachern	Dec 18, 1965–July 5, 1968
Hon John C. Munro	July 5, 1968–

B. DEPUTY MINISTERS

Dr John A. Amyot	1919–1932
Dr Robert E. Wodehouse	1932–1944
Dr Brock Chisholm (Health)	1944–1946
G.F. Davidson (Welfare)	1944–1960
Dr D.G.W. Cameron (Health)	1946–1965
Joseph W. Willard (Welfare)	1960–
Dr John N. Crawford (Health)	1965–1970
Dr J. Maurice LeClair (Health)	1970–

Canadian Hospital (Council) Association

Presidents
1931–1935 F.W. Routley, MD

1935–1937 W.R. Chenoweth
1937–1939 Father Geo. Verreault
1939–1945 George F. Stephens, MD
1945–1949 Arthur J. Swanson
1949–1951 R. Fraser-Armstrong

1951–1953 O.C. Trainer, MD

1953–1955 A.C. McGugan, MD

1955–1957 J. Gilbert Turner, MD
1959   D.F.W. Porter, MD
1959–1961 Stanley W. Martin
1961–1963 Judge N.V. Buchanan
1963–1965 A.H. Westbury
1965–1966 C.E. Barton

1966–1968 Chaiker Abbis, QC
1968–1969 R. Alan Hay

Executive Directors
G. Harvey Agnew, MD
(1931–July 1950)

L.O. Bradley, MD
(July 1950–July 1951)
Arnold J. Swanson, MD
(Sept 1951–Sept 1954)
W. Douglas Piercey, MD
(Oct 1954–1965)

George McCracken
Asst Director Finance,
acting Executive Director
(Nov 1965–July 1966)

B.L.P. Brosseau, MD
(1966–

1969–1970 L.R. Adshead
1970–1971 Gaston Rodrique, MD
1971–1972 Wm A. Holland
1972–1973 Judge E.N. Hughes

NOTE The executive officer was called 'secretary' or 'executive secretary' until September 1954; thereafter, he was known as 'executive director.'

APPENDIX D

Charter CHA Members

Those in attendance at the inaugural meeting of the Canadian Hospital Council, 1931, in Toronto:

DELEGATES AND ALTERNATES
Hospital Association of Nova Scotia and Prince Edward Island
L.D. Currie, Glace Bay, Nova Scotia
Rev H.G. Wright, Inverness, Nova Scotia
Maritime Conference of the Catholic Hospital Association
Mother Audet, Campbellton, New Brunswick
Sister Beatrice, Antigonish, Nova Scotia (alternate for Mother Ignatius)
Father Robert J. Williams, Chatham, New Brunswick
New Brunswick Hospital Association
Miss A.J. MacMaster, Moncton, New Brunswick
Dr R.J. Collins, Saint John, New Brunswick
Montreal Hospital Council
Dr A.L.C. Gilday, Montreal, Quebec
J.H. Roy, Montreal, Quebec (alternate for Dr L.A. Lessard)
W.R. Chenoweth, Montreal, Quebec
Ontario Hospital Association
Dr John Ferguson, Toronto, Ontario
Dr Fred W. Routley, Toronto, Ontario
Ontario Conference of the Catholic Hospital Association
Rev Wilfred Smith, Toronto, Ontario
Rev Sister St Elizabeth, Toronto, Ontario
Rev Sister Margaret, Toronto, Ontario (alternate)

Manitoba Hospital Association
Dr George F. Stephens, Winnipeg, Manitoba
Dr Gerald S. Williams, Winnipeg, Manitoba
Saskatchewan Hospital Association
Dr S.R.D. Hewitt, Regina, Saskatchewan
Alberta Hospital Association
Dr R.T. Washburn, Edmonton, Alberta
Dr A.F. Anderson, Edmonton, Alberta
British Columbia Hospital Association
Dr A.K. Haywood, Vancouver, British Columbia (observing delegate)
Department of Hospital Service, Canadian Medical Association
Dr G. Harvey Agnew, Toronto

SPECIAL INVITED DELEGATES
Dr W.J. Dobbie, Hospital for Consumptives, Weston, Ontario (Tuberculosis Hospitals)
Dr R.E. Wodehouse, Ottawa, Deputy Minister, Department of Pensions and National Health
Dr Ross Miller, Director of Medical Services, Department of Pensions and National Health
Dr B.T. McGhie, Director of Hospital Services, Province of Ontario

OBSERVERS
Frank D. Reville, President-elect, OHA
Dr T.C. Routley, General Secretary, CMA
Rev Alphonse Schwitalla, St Louis, Missouri, President, Catholic Hospital Association of United States and Canada
Miss E.M. McKee, Superintendent, Brantford General Hospital
A.J. Swanson, Superintendent, Toronto Western Hospital
Rev Mother Allaire, Grey Nunnery, Montreal
Miss Priscilla Campbell, Superintendent, Chatham Hospital, Chatham, Ontario
Ray Kneifl, Editor, *Hospital Progress*, St Louis, Missouri
Miss Ruth C. Wilson, Assistant Superintendent, Moncton City Hospital
Miss G.M. Meharg, Librarian, Department of Hospital Services, CMA
Sister Margaret, Secretary, Ontario Conference of the Catholic Hospital Association (listed as alternate above)
J.C. MacKenzie, Superintendent of the Montreal General Hospital
Mary Burcher, Editor, *Canadian Hospital*

INITIAL OFFICERS OF THE CANADIAN HOSPITAL
COUNCIL

Honorary President   Hon R.B. Bennett, Prime Minister of Canada
Honorary Vice-President   Hon Dr Murray MacLaren
President   Dr F.W. Routley
First Vice-President   W.R. Chenoweth
Second Vice-President   Rev Mother Audet
Secretary-Treasurer   Dr G. Harvey Agnew
Executive Committee F.W. Routley, W.R. Chenoweth, George Stephens, L.D. Currie, G. Harvey Agnew

CHA Second Meeting

Delegates to the second meeting of the Canadian Hospital Council in Winnipeg, 1933:
Hospital Association of Nova Scotia and Prince Edward Island
L.D. Currie, Glace Bay, Nova Scotia
Rev H.G. Wright, Inverness, Nova Scotia
New Brunswick Hospital Association
Dr R.J. Collins, Saint John, New Brunswick
Miss A.J. MacMaster, Moncton, New Brunswick
Maritime Conference of the Catholic Hospital Association
Rev Mother Audet, Campbelltown, New Brunswick
Rev Dr R.J. Williams, Chatham, New Brunswick
Rev Mother Ignatius, Antigonish, Nova Scotia
Rev Sister Beatrice, Antigonish, Nova Scotia (alternate)
Montreal Hospital Council
Dr A.L.C. Gilday, Montreal
Dr L.A. Lessard, Montreal
J.H. Roy, Montreal (alternate)
W.R. Chenoweth, Montreal (alternate)
L'Association des Hôpitaux de la Province de Québec
Rev Monseignor Grandbois
Rev Father Durocher
Ontario Hospital Association
Dr F.W. Routley, Toronto
Dr John Ferguson, Toronto
Ontario Conference of the Catholic Hospital Association
Rev Wilfred Smith, Toronto

Rev Sister St Elizabeth, London
Rev Sister Campion, Kingston (alternate)
Rev Sister Margaret, Toronto
Manitoba Hospital Association
Dr G.F. Stephens, Winnipeg
Dr G.S. Williams, Winnipeg
Saskatchewan Hospital Association
Leonard Shaw, Saskatoon
R.T. Graham, Swift Current
S.H. Curran, Yorkton
Alberta Hospital Association
Dr R.T. Washburn, University Hospital, Edmonton
Dr A.F. Anderson, Edmonton
Prairie Provinces Conference of the Catholic Hospital Association
Rev H. Bourque, St Boniface
Rev Mother Leberge, Edmonton
Sister Mary of Jesus, Winnipeg (alternate)
British Columbia Hospital Association
J.M. Coady, Vancouver
J.H. McVety, Vancouver
Department of Hospital Services of the Canadian Medical Association
Dr A.K. Haywood, Vancouver
Dr G.H. Agnew, Toronto
Associate Members
Department of Pensions and National Health: Dr Ross Miller
Province of Prince Edward Island: Hon W.J.P. MacMillan, Minister of Education and Public Health
Province of New Brunswick: Dr William Warwick, Chief Medical Officer
Province of Quebec: Dr Alphonse Lessard, Director of Public Charities
Province of Ontario: Dr B.T. McGhie, Director of Hospital Services
Province of Manitoba: Dr F.W. Jackson, Deputy Minister of Health
Province of Saskatchewan: Dr F.C. Middleton, Deputy Minister of Health
Province of Alberta: Dr E.A. Braithwaite, Inspector of Hospitals
Province of British Columbia: P. de N. Walker, Deputy Provincial Secretary

OFFICERS ELECTED AT 1933 MEETING
President Dr F.W. Routley
First Vice-President W.R. Chenoweth
Second Vice-President Rev Mother Allaire
Secretary-Treasurer Dr G. Harvey Agnew
Executive Committee Above, with Leonard Shaw and J.M. Coady

Catholic Hospital Association of Canada[1]

Presidents	Executive Directors
1943–1945 Mother M. Berthe Dorais St Boniface	
1945–1952 Rev H.L. Bertrand, sj Montreal	
1952–1953 Rev John Fullerton, sj, Toronto	Rev Henri Legare
1953–1954 Rt Rev Victorin Germain Quebec	(1952–1956)
1955–1956 Rev J.A. Leahy Vancouver	Rev Francis J. Smyth (1956–1958)
1957–1958 Rev Joseph B. Nearing Sydney Mines, Nova Scotia	
1959–1960 Rev Raymond Durocher Winnipeg	Rev A.L.M. Danis (1958–1967)
1961–1962 Mother Berthe Dorais Montreal	
1963 Rev F.J. Smyth Antigonish, Nova Scotia	
1964–1965 Rev C.S. Godin Estevan, Saskatchewan	
1966–1967 Rt Rev Edgar Godin Bathurst, New Brunswick	Rev Maurice Dussault (1967–1972)

1 The association was known as the Catholic Hospital Council of Canada prior to 1954.

1968	Rev Sister M. Honora	
	Toronto	
1969	Lucien Lacoste	
	Montreal	
1970	Jean-Marc Daoust	
	Montreal	
1971	Rev Norman Andries	
	Saskatchewan	
1972	Maj J.J.H. Connors	Rev Norman Andries
	Manitoba	(1972–)
1973	Dr E.G.Q. Van Tilburg	
	New Brunswick	

CHAC Purposes and objects

The following is extracted from the Constitution and By-Laws of the Catholic Hospital Association of Canada/Association des Hôpitaux Catholiques du Canada:

PURPOSES AND OBJECTS OF THE ASSOCIATION

A

To promote and realize a more efficacious programme for the spiritual and corporal care of the sick, infirm and aged in those institution in Canada which are administered or managed by a Roman Catholic religious organization of Sisters and Brothers or by any one or group of lay persons duly approved by Roman Catholic ecclesiastical authority;

B

to foster higher ideals in the religious, moral, medical, nursing, educational, social and all other phases of hospital and nursing endeavour and other consistent purposes especially relating to the Catholic hospitals and schools of nursing in Canada;

C

to correlate and co-ordinate the activities of the various Catholic hospital organizations to above-mentioned ends;

D

to represent its members in those matters of general or national interest which concern their welfare;

E

to undertake the study of the philosophy and the religious life of hospitals, their legislation, organization, finance, construction, medical staff, nursing staff and education, the relationship of the hospital to federal, provincial and municipal governments and the general public, and such subjects as affect the administration of hospitals;

F

to co-operate with governments, other hospital organizations and any other body in promoting public health and welfare and the improvement of hospitals generally;

G

to foster and promote periodic conventions, study weeks, courses in hospital administration, the publication of books, magazines, pamphlets and other types of literature, and other means to best achieve the objectives herein set forth;

H

to accept financial or other forms of assistance for the Corporation from sources outside its membership for the purpose of furthering the objects of the Corporation.

Canadian ACHA Charter Fellows

The following Canadians (and former Canadians active in the hospital field in the United States) were elected to charter fellowship in the American College of Hospital Administrators.

Honorary Charter Fellows
Dr G. Harvey Agnew, Toronto
Dr Malcom T. MacEachern, Vancouver and Chicago
Charter Fellows
Chester J. Decker, Toronto
Dr Alfred K. Haywood, Montreal and Vancouver
Dr S.R.D. Hewitt, Regina and Saint John, NB
Muriel McKee (Mrs C.C. Carris), Brantford, Ontario
Henry Rowland, Toronto
Dr George F. Stephens, Winnipeg and Montreal
Arthur J. Swanson, Toronto
Former Canadians
E. Muriel Anscombe, St Louis
Mabel Marr, Philadelphia
Dr Allan Craig, Chicago and New York
Thomas T. Murray, New York
Dr Donald C. Smelzer, Philadelphia
Dr Peter D. Ward, Minneapolis

APPENDIX I

Canadian College of Health Service Executives Initial Executive Committee

President Dr Leonard O. Bradley, Toronto
First Vice-President L.R. Adshead, Calgary
Second Vice-President W.R. Slatkoff, Montreal
Secretary-Treasurer R.E. McDermitt, Regina
Assistant Secretary E.N. Stefanuk, Toronto
Regional Directors:
F.S. Whittington, British Columbia, Alberta, Northwest Territories
John Carter, Saskatchewan, Manitoba
Kenneth E. Box, Ontario
Sister Bernadette Poirer, Quebec
H.K. Frowd, Atlantic Provinces
R.D. Moore, Canadian Hospital Association

Index

276 Index